# AQUATIC TOXICOLOGY

## VOLUME 1

# Aquatic Toxicology

## *Volume 1*

Editor

### Lavern J. Weber, Ph.D.
*Director*
*Marine Science Center*
*Oregon State University*
*Newport, Oregon*

Raven Press ■ New York

**Raven Press, 1140 Avenue of the Americas, New York, New York 10036**

Made in the United States of America

**Library of Congress Cataloging in Publication Data**
Main entry under title:

Aquatic toxicology.

    Includes index.
    1. Aquatic organisms—Effect of water pollution
on.    2. Water—Pollution—Toxicology.    3. Water
quality bioassay.    I. Weber, Lavern J. [DNLM:
1. Toxicology—Period.    2. Water pollutants—
Toxicity—Period. W1 AQ927]
QH545.W3A65    574.2′4    81–23474
ISBN 0–89004–439–2 (V. 1)    AACR2

Great care has been taken to maintain the accuracy of the information contained in the volume. However, Raven Press cannot be held responsible for errors or for any consequences arising from the use of the information contained herein.

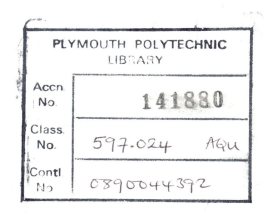

# Preface

During the past two decades of environmental concern, there has been increasing interest in the impact of physical and chemical environmental changes to man and all other biological organisms. Studies on the effects of environmental perturbations have ranged from broad ecological investigations to studies on individual species. Our understanding of the influence of these changes on individual aquatic organisms has benefited from the existence of a broad knowledge base of physiology, biochemistry, pharmacology, and toxicology of terrestrial animals, especially mammals. By the early 1980s, the accumulated information on the responses of aquatic organisms to changes in their physical environment was extensive enough to justify a series of reviews of the state of this knowledge. *Aquatic Toxicology* provides these reviews.

This first volume covers the cardiovascular system and the many complexities that can be examined in the various fishes used in cardiovascular toxicology. The hepatic system is reviewed at the organ function level and then carried into a very specific mixed-function oxidase induction system in another chapter. One chapter is devoted to chemical carcinogenesis in fish because of the relative sensitivity of a fish model system for carcinogenesis.

Future volumes will include chapters on the respiratory system, renal system, nervous system, and specific toxicants, such as cyanide. They will also cover the areas of toxicological and comparative biomedical studies of aquatic invertebrates

From an organizational standpoint, *Aquatic Toxicology* proceeds from the general to the specific. First to be examined is whole animal toxicology with emphasis on routes of administration and exposure to toxicants of concern in the environment. Next, the organ system level of organization is considered with reviews of specific functional organ toxicity. Toxicological studies at the operational level are reviewed next. By operational, we refer to the effects that a toxicant has on very specific physiological and biochemical systems, such as enzymes, receptors, and membranes. Specific classes of toxicants will be reviewed in future volumes.

Although this text focuses primarily on aquatic animals, analogies to mammalian systems are included for comparison. Discrepancies of experimental conditions and the problems with the numerous species involved in the aquatic environment are indicated. The many problems of water quality conditions, including pH, temperature, hardness, alkalinity, and salt concentrations found in various areas are discussed.

The purpose of this book is to review the various organ systems and toxicological problems for investigators in the field and to cover the basics of the field for the biologist and biomedical researcher who intend to use aquatic organisms for model systems or very specific studies. It is intended to help educate the reader about the many peculiarities of the species involved. There are in excess of 20,000 species of fish, with life styles, habitats, morphology, and physiology more diverse within the fishes than in the most unusual species of mammals. An effort has been made to delineate many of these differences and the consequent problems in physiological, biochemical, pharmacological, and toxicological studies caused by this diversity.

These toxicological reviews cover whole animal, physiological, pharmacological, and biochemical levels of investigation of aquatic organisms. This volume will be of interest to all who utilize aquatic organisms in biomedical research of a toxicological nature.

*Lavern J. Weber*

# Acknowledgment

This study was supported in part by the Marine and Freshwater Biomedical Core Center Grant, NIEHS ES01926.

# Contents

*ix*

# Contributors

**C. R. Elcombe.** *Central Toxicology Laboratory, Imperial Chemical Industries, Macclesfield, Cheshire, England*

**William H. Gingerich.** *National Fishery Research Laboratory, La Crosse, Wisconsin 54601*

**Jerry D. Hendricks.** *Department of Food Science and Technology, Oregon State University, Corvallis, Oregon 97331*

**John F. Klaverkamp.** *Fisheries and Oceans Canada Freshwater Institute, Winnipeg, Manitoba, Canada R3T 2N6*

**John J. Lech.** *Department of Pharmacology and Toxicology, The Medical College of Wisconsin, Milwaukee, Wisconsin 53226 and The Great Lakes Research Facility, University of Wisconsin, Milwaukee, Wisconsin 53201*

**Mary Jo Vodicnik.** *Department of Pharmacology and Toxicology, The Medical College of Wisconsin, Milwaukee, Wisconsin 53226 and The Great Lakes Research Facility, University of Wisconsin, Milwaukee, Wisconsin 53201*

*Aquatic Toxicology*, edited by Lavern J. Weber,
Raven Press, New York © 1982.

# The Physiological Pharmacology and Toxicology of Fish Cardiovascular Systems

J. F. Klaverkamp

*Fisheries and Oceans Canada, Freshwater Institute,
Winnipeg, Manitoba, Canada R3T 2N6*

This chapter is written for research students and other investigators who have a fundamental understanding of the pharmacology and physiology of mammalian cardiovascular systems and of fish cardiovascular anatomy, and who have an interest in initiating research on the pharmacology and toxicology of fish cardiovascular systems. It must be emphasized at the onset that there are more species of fish than there are species in all the other vertebrate classes combined; and fish have a great diversity of structure, reflecting the fact that the origins of different groups extend back from the Cretaceous to the Devonian. The broad definitions of pharmacology, as the study of the effects of chemicals on the function of these systems, and of toxicology, as investigations directed to those effects considered adverse to the organism, have been used (100).

After a brief introduction on fish cardiovascular structure and dynamics, with emphasis on the major pre- and postgill vasculature, attention is focused on a historical review of classic pharmacological analyses of cardiovascular responses to humoral compounds and neurotransmitters and, finally, on the use of fish cardiovascular responses in aquatic toxicology programs. Discussions of fish cardiovascular pharmacology have been limited to brief summaries in articles on fish physiology (114,140,158,159). A thorough review of this area of pharmacology is required, however, for at least two reasons. First, understanding the nature and magnitude of inherent

*1*

responses of physiological systems to chemicals is essential for providing accurate interpretation of results in toxicology. Second, methods and procedures developed in pharmacological analyses frequently guide the selection of approaches in toxicological investigations. Consequently, an appreciation of the types of responses and available approaches will assist the investigator who is initiating research in this area.

Comprehensive references are available for the reader interested in the broader aspects of fish cardiovascular physiology (140,158); in specialized areas, such as microcirculation (159); in processes involving the gill, such as gas exchange (78,141,193), acid-base balance (1,193), and osmoregulation (108); in the innervation of fish cardiovascular systems (24,157,159); and in comparative cardiorespiratory physiology of nonmammalian vertebrates (193).

## CARDIOVASCULAR STRUCTURE AND DYNAMICS

With the exception of certain cyclostomes and air-breathing fish, there is a general conformity of structure in fish cardiovascular systems. The heart is divided into four chambers located in series in the order of the sinus venosus, atrium, ventricle, and conus arteriosus or, in teleost fish, the bulbus arteriosus. The electrocardiogram may exhibit as many as four deflections, one preceding the contraction of each of the four chambers (G. H. Satchell, *personal communication*). In most fish, the pacemaker site is in the sinus venosus (156), usually at the sinoatrial valve (71). The heart pumps venous blood and is located in a pericardium, which is generally rigid in elasmobranchs and flexible in teleosts (158). Flow is kept unidirectional by valves located at the sinoatrial and atrioventricular openings and at the junction of the ventricle and the conus or the bulbus. From the heart, blood is passed in sequence to the ventral aorta, with some alternative pathways through the branchial (gill) circulation for oxygenation, and then into the dorsal aorta. Alternative pathways to blood flowing through the branchial vasculature include a hypobranchial circulation including the pseudobranch, a

filamental circulation from the efferent filament arteries, and a nutritive circulation to the gill arch and interbranchial septum (170).
From the dorsal aorta, which is the major postgill arterial vessel,
blood goes to either the hepatic, the systemic and intestinal, or the
renal capillary system. Venous blood finally collects in the sinus
venosus and then returns to the heart. The heart pumps only venous
blood and the coronary arteries arise, not from the aorta close to
the valves, as in mammals, but from the efferent gill arteries that
carry oxygenated blood. For a schematic representation of a salmonid heart and associated vasculature, see Fig. 1.

There are two basic variations to this general scheme. Hagfish
have accessory hearts in their circulatory systems, as well as a larger
blood volume and lower blood pressure (140). Lungfish have a
pulmonary circulation and a partial separation of oxygenated and
deoxygenated blood in their hearts (80).

The rest of this section will emphasize the physiology and structure of large blood vessels, since this has been a neglected area in
recent reviews. A recent chapter by Satchell (159) provides a thorough review of capillary types and gill microcirculation. Detailed

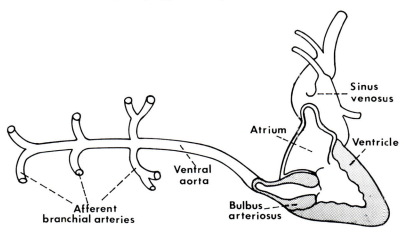

**FIG. 1.** A schematic representation of a salmonid heart and associated
vasculature.

descriptions of the mechanical and electrical events of the cardiac cycle and other aspects of cardiac physiology have been presented in texts of fish physiology (140,158).

The bulbus arteriosus does not contain cardiac muscle or contract actively in sequence with the heart. It has been referred to by Satchell (158) as the "intrapericardial portion of the ventral aorta that balloons out to form [a] thick-walled onion-shaped chamber." Johansen (78) has called the bulbus "a swelling at the base of the heart, composed of arterial smooth muscle and elastic tissue." Regarding the distensibility of the tissue, Lansing (98) has remarked that "the organ is highly elastic, more so than any biological material previously encountered." Recent investigations on the innervation and vascularization of this organ have demonstrated the typical three layers found in vasculature, namely, the adventitia, media, and intima, and the presence of innervated smooth muscle cells within the media (192).

The bulbus arteriosus has been reported to act as an elastic reservoir to dampen the rise and fall of blood pressure as well as the fluctuations in flow rate (77). The crucial role of the tissue is not only to protect the gill capillaries from the pressure fluctuations, but to extend positive aortic flow through a larger portion of the cardiac cycle (78,140,158). Johansen (77) has reported that positive aortic flow exists in the ventral aorta of the cod for more than three-quarters of the cardiac cycle, whereas in mammals it is present for less than one-third. The importance of this flow prolongation is particularly significant when the relatively low heart rate of fish is considered: 30 beats/min in the cod (77), 21 in the carp (58), 32 in the Japanese eel, 46 in the rainbow trout (75), and 30 in largemouth bass (150).

Another function of the bulbus related to its incorporation into the pericardium and its intricate anatomical relationship with the atrium has been suggested (112,113). The bulbus is directly below the atrium, which is grooved on its ventral surface, and the two fit precisely together, emptying and filling reciprocally. From this arrangement, the bulbus modulates atrial activity and prevents the development of negative pressure within the pericardium (Holst, 1969 in ref. 158).

In a report discussing arterial system capacitance and capillary bed resistance in model mammalian circulatory system design, Taylor (184) has pointed out the good correlation of vascular system function with the mechanical properties of the tissue. Satchell (158) has extended circulatory system model designing to fish, which have two arterial systems in series, both distal from an intermittent pump action and placed on either side of a gill capillary bed. To achieve an even flow through this capillary resistance, Satchell has pointed out the requirements of having a diminished capacitance in the arterial system distal from the gills (dorsal aorta) and a large smoothing capacitance in the arterial system between the heart and the gills (ventral aorta). In other words, the model fish circulatory system should and, in fact, does have a large, compliant ventral aorta and a rigid, nondistensible dorsal aorta.

Additional studies on the histology and elastic modulus (the ratio of elastic tension developed to the amount of deformation that elicited it) support these functional characteristics in mammals and fish. Determinations of the elastic modulus in mammals have shown that vessels with a large ratio are rich in collagen, low in elastin, and have rather nondistensible walls, whereas vessels with low values are dominated by elastin and are easily distensible (153,184). These studies have also shown that elastin fibers are recruited by a very slight stretching of the wall and that the less extensible collagen is not stretched until the vessel is largely distended. Similar studies in sharks (Lander, 1964 and Learoyd, 1963 both cited in ref. 158) have shown that there is a gradient of diminishing elastin content from the proximal end of the ventral aorta through the afferent and efferent arteries up to the dorsal aorta. From the proximal to the distal end, the dorsal aorta is consistently low in elastin (9%) (mg/100 mg dried fat-free tissue × 100) and high in collagen (69%) (Lander, 1964 cited in ref. 158). The average elastin content in the ventral aorta was 31%, whereas collagen was 46%. Thus, the ventral aorta, which contains about three times more elastin than the dorsal aorta, is also relatively high in collagen. Values for rabbit thoracic aorta are 45 to 50% elastin and 20 to 25% collagen (184).

The ventral aorta of sharks consists of the typical three layers of tissue found in the vertebrate arterial wall (Lander, 1964 cited in ref. 158). The adventitia and media together constitute about one-eighth of the total wall thickness and are largely made up of collagen. The media is largely made up of circularly arranged elastin fibers with smooth muscle cells in between. By contrast, the adventitia of the dorsal aorta of the shark constitutes three-fourths of the total wall thickness and is extremely collagenous. There is no separate intimal layer and the remaining one-fourth is made up of the media layer, which has a twofold higher proportion of elastin than the whole wall. The dorsal aorta, which runs below and is attached to the spinal column, is not a symmetrical tubular vessel. The vessel wall is much thinner on the side facing the ventral surface of the vertebrae, and there is only a small amount of collagenous tissue with no circular muscle fiber in this region. The adventitia of the ventral surface of the dorsal aorta is "extended laterally to form a girdle of strands that lashes the aorta to the vertebrae" (158). Similar anatomical arrangements and histological features of the ventral and dorsal aortae have been described for the carp (44).

Investigations using perfused isolated trunk (201) and intact perfused gill (195) preparations from rainbow trout have demonstrated the large extent of passive distensibility in systemic and branchial circulations. Branchial vascular resistance is altered much more effectively by changing dorsal aortic pressure than by changing ventral aortic pressure. Autoregulatory mechanisms may also affect this resistance. The authors point out that there is considerable distensibility in the branchial vasculature, but that the systemic vascular resistance is more distensible at normal levels of blood pressure. This difference in distensibility may be less than these studies indicate, since a perfused head preparation with simulated normal dorsal aortic blood pressure was used to evaluate branchial vascular distensibility. Smith (170) described these branchial preparations as unaccountably sensitive to changes in outflow pressure and suggests that they are subject to disrupted flow rates.

## THE PHYSIOLOGICAL PHARMACOLOGY OF FISH CARDIOVASCULAR SYSTEMS

As stated at the beginning of this chapter, knowledge of procedures used in pharmacology guides selection of approaches to toxicological investigations, especially those that are directed to understanding basic mechanisms of action. In order to focus attention on the procedures used to assess cardiovascular function in intact fish and to investigate control mechanisms of the major components of the system, this section is organized into four general subtopics. Described are studies on intact cardiovascular systems, isolated heart preparations, isolated gill preparations, and isolated vascular preparations. Within each subtopic, there is discussion of the relative effects of classes of neuronal and humoral compounds, in order to understand the pharmacological nature and magnitude of inherent responses in a given preparation.

### Intact Cardiovascular Preparations

*Experimental Design and Procedures*

There has been considerable variation in experimental design and procedures since the first comprehensive study of pharmacological responses in the cardiovascular system of intact fish was conducted by MacKay (107). Skates weighing from 4 to 5 kg were immobilized by spinal cord transection or barbiturate anesthesia, and the ventral aorta was cannulated to record blood pressure. Drugs were injected into the lateral vein leading directly to the heart or into the gastric vein to observe the effects of hepatic circulation.

In the year subsequent to MacKay's report, the first major modification in surgical and cannulating procedures was presented (202). In addition to recording ventral aortic blood pressure from one of the branchial arteries, these workers cannulated the celiac artery and were able to monitor dorsal aortic blood pressure. This modification enabled them to observe changes in branchial as well as systemic vascular resistance. Also, this modification did not alter the interpretation of the observations of the cardiac parameters measured by McKay (107), so a description of more cardiovascular responses of the intact system could be made.

In the years following these two pioneering reports, there have been many variations in experimental procedures. As in mammalian cardiovascular pharmacology, there has been continual application of new and improved technology. There have been major differences in surgical procedures, vasculature cannulated, approaches to restraint and anesthesia, expression of dosage, route of drug administration, and presentation of data.

Simultaneous recording of pre- and postbranchial blood pressures have increased the understanding of the control and regulation of branchial vascular resistance. Techniques for obtaining prebranchial blood pressure include the cannulation of the ventral aorta (15,86,114,177,195); of one of the afferent branchial ateries (20,79,146,189); of the bulbus arteriosus (32,33); and of one of the cardiac chambers (33). Postbranchial blood pressures have been obtained by direct cannulation of the dorsal aorta (15,33,195) or by cannulation of one of the major arteries branching from the dorsal aorta (32,79,113,146,177,189,195).

In other studies, blood pressure from only one vessel was recorded. Cannulation sites included the ventral aorta (194), the bulbus arteriosus (31,34), an afferent branchial artery (20), the caudal portion of the dorsal aorta (163,164,165,187), one of its branches (36,82,128), or an anterior section of the dorsal aorta (144,171).

Heart rate can easily be determined from blood pressure tracings and from electrocardiogram records (75,116,128,137,139). Cardiac output has been determined by indirect dilution methods (58,75,115), by direct measurements on the excised ventricle (60), and, more recently, by direct measurements on intact, functioning systems using a flow-probe around the major prebranchial vasculature (33,86,195). Electromagnetic probes have also been used to measure blood flow through the celiac artery, one of the major branches of the dorsal aorta (61).

In addition to *in vivo* studies, the effects of drugs on vascular resistance have been investigated by perfusion experiments on vascular segments *in situ*. Perfusion of the systemic vasculature has been conducted through the dorsal aorta (87,146,201,197,199) or one of its branches (31,34,59), while the branchial vasculature has been perfused through the ventral aorta (146,195,197) and the bulbus arteriosus (51). The perfused branchial and systemic preparations will be discussed in the isolated gill and isolated vasculature sections, respectively.

An artificially ventilated, perfused whole rainbow trout preparation has recently been described (200). These investigators perfused the anterior end of the sectioned ventral aorta and collected the venous effluent from the posterior end. Kent and Pierce (86) have used similar auto- and pump-perfused preparations of the dogfish shark.

There have also been differences reported in the intravascular route of administration of the drugs. These include intravenous injections that either lead directly to the heart (22,33,37,86, 107,113,202), or travel first through a portal circulation (26,31,32,107, 128,144,161,163,164,165,177,187,189,195). Intraarterial injections have also been used to administer drugs (79,82,86,146,171,194).

*Pharmacology*

*Responses to Adrenergic and Cholinergic Agents*

MacKay (107) observed that epinephrine (Epi) produces a marked, dose-related increase in ventral aortic blood pressure of the skate, which begins after a latent period of ½ to 1 min and reaches a maximum several min later. The duration of the response is long; a dose of 0.1 mg in a 4 kg skate lasts 1 to 2-½ hr. Epi increases the force of cardiac contraction while the rate decreases; injection through the hepatic circulation does not diminish the responses. Fish severely stressed by capture do not respond to Epi unless they rest for several days. The negative chronotropic response to Epi was later found to be part of a reflex mechanism mediated by the vagus nerve (114).

MacKay reasoned that since sympathetic innervation is not present, the direct effect of Epi on the heart is not very marked, and the duration of action is long, the "point of action of adrenalin on the blood vessels may be directly on the muscles of the arteries or on the receptor substance in them, which is developed at this special evolutionary stage but which is not yet connected by the sympathetic nervous system to the central nervous system" (107).

In the decades following MacKay's work, many other investigators concluded that a sympathetic nerve supply to the heart of fish is lacking (see review by Burnstock, ref. 16). More recent research has demonstrated the presence of adrenergic innervation in the teleost heart (22,23,54,65) and vasculature (65,66,120, 171,185,192,196), although this innervation is very sparse or lacking in the cardiovascular systems of elasmobranchs (57,123), such as MacKay's skates (107). Burnstock (17) has described sympathetic adrenergic nerves as a "relatively recent evolutionary advance" and has stated that "a higher proportion of sympathetic nerves in lower vertebrates is cholinergic than in mammals." Embryological investigations on autonomic nervous system development also support the view that cholinergic innervation is "phylogenetically more primitive" than adrenergic innervation in regulating cardiovascular systems (14).

Concentrations, expressed in $\mu g/100$ ml, of Epi and norepinephrine (NE), up to 36 and 20, respectively, have been observed in plasma from "stressed" teleost fish, while concentrations of 0.5 and 0.3, respectively, were usually observed in "resting" fish (117,121,134). Using a radioenzymatic technique, Butler et al. (20) have found concentrations, again expressed in $\mu g/100$ ml, of Epi and NE up to 0.34 and 1.68, respectively, in plasma from hypoxia-stressed dogfish (elasmobranch), and concentrations of 0.08 and 0.09, respectively, in normoxic fish. While release of catecholamines from adrenergic nerves may contribute to all of these concentrations (22,170), the major source of them is probably from chromaffin tissue surrounding the postcardinal vein in the head kidney (65,117,121,158,159).

Since the early work of McWilliam on mechanisms of cardio-vascular control in the eel (111), the dominance of cholinergic mechanisms, especially on the heart, has been well documented (16,158). There is, however, some controversy about the significance of vagal tone on heart rate in resting fish (22,137,140,177). Recent investigations have provided insight into the site of action of acetylcholine in teleost gills (170). There are some apparent anomalies relative to mammalian pharmacology; for example, in some fish, phenoxybenzamine is more effective than atropine in blocking cholinergic responses (17).

The pronounced and dose-related vasopressor response produced by Epi in the skate (107) has also been reported in other elasmo-branch species (15,26,86,163,165,202), in teleost species (32,33,36,51,144,146,163,177), and in the lungfish (82). Epi and NE increase resistance in the perfused systemic vasculature of hagfish, although no effects were observed in the intact circulation (146).

Some authors have commented on the similarity of NE to Epi, but have done so in a qualitative, rather than a quantitative, fashion (82,113,146,164). NE has been described as being two to three times less potent than Epi in eliciting a pressor response in the cat shark and catfish (163). Using perfused preparations, Wood (197,198) has concluded that Epi is more potent than NE in the systemic vasculature, but that there is a reversal of this potency ranking in the gills. While the branchial vasculature is more sensitive to these catecholamines than the systemic (195,197,201), the effects of catecholamines on systemic vasculature may be more important in regulating resistance of intact systems than their effects on branchial vasculature (51).

The effects of other catecholamines have also been investigated on intact preparations. Isoproterenol (Isop) produces a dorsal aortic depressor response in two species of shark (164), and in the lungfish (82). In the cod (177) and eel (33), Isop produces a decrease in pre- and postbranchial blood pressure, but has little effect on heart rate. Phenylephrine produces an increase in pre- and postbranchial blood pressures with a decrease in heart rate of the cod (177). Dopamine has no effects on blood pressure but produces a decrease in heart rate of the cod (33).

Small doses of Epi in intact fish have little effect on heart rate, whereas larger doses, for example, 5 μg/kg in the cod, generally produce bradycardia (15,165,177,202). This Epi-induced decrease in heart rate is blocked by atropine (33,144) and hyoscine (177), and is a reflex mechanism mediated by cholinergic mechanisms of the vagus nerve. It is temperature dependent in the carp, since a decrease in heart rate was observed from 1°C to 8°C and an increase was observed from 9°C to 20°C (97).

Tachyphylaxis, the failure of subsequent doses of a chemical to produce a response regardless of concentration, resulting from high doses of catecholamines has been observed with the pressor response to Epi and with the depressor response to Isop (100,113,164,165,202). Tachyphylaxis has also been observed in the pressor response of tyramine in the eel (33).

Comprehensive investigations utilizing pharmacological blockers, neurotransmitter releasers, or synthesis inhibitors in intact cardiovascular systems have been conducted in coho and sockeye salmon (144), rainbow trout (195), cod (177,189), eel (33,51,52), dogfish shark (26), and goldfish (22). After administration of atropine, Epi does not produce a decreased heart rate in salmon and an augmentation of the dorsal aortic pressor response is exhibited (144). Phenoxybenzamine blocks the pressor effects of Epi and occasionally produces an increase in heart rate. The β-adrenergic blockers dichloroisoproterenol and propranolol produce decreases in dorsal aortic blood pressure and heart rate but have little effect on the pressor response to Epi.

In the eel, catecholamines, with a relative potency of NE > Epi >> Isop, increase cardiac contractile force by acting on α-adrenergic receptors, since it can be blocked by phentolamine but not by propranolol (33). Epi produces a decrease in transbranchial pressure that is blocked by propranolol, indicating the presence of β-adrenergic receptors in branchial vasculature. Pressor effects produced by Epi and NE in the systemic circulation are blocked by phentolamine and phenoxybenzamine, and the depressor effects produced by Isop are abolished by propranolol. These responses demonstrate the presence of α- and β-adrenergic receptors in eel vasculature. Both of these receptors are also found in dogfish shark vasculature (28). While α- and β-adrenergic receptors are found in eel heart, other species of teleosts demonstrate considerable variation in adrenergic receptor type in their hearts (22,52).

As in salmon heart, there are β-adrenergic receptors controlling heart rate in cod, since propranolol produces a decrease in heart rate (143,177,189). Systemic pressor effects produced by Epi, NE, and phenylephrine are blocked by yohimbine, indicating the presence of α-adrenergic receptors. Experiments using 6-hydroxydopamine and reserpine have been conducted to evaluate the role of adrenergic nerves innervating the heart and vasculature and of circulating catecholamines released, for example, from chromaffin tissue in the head kidney (121,189). The investigators have concluded that gill vessels play a little role in regulating systemic blood pressure and that "adrenergic tonus" affecting heart rate and blood pressure is primarily produced by circulating catecholamines rather than adrenergic innervation (177,189). The use of a perfused head kidney and heart preparation from the cod has also demonstrated that the release of catecholamines from chromaffin tissue plays an important role in regulating the heart (65).

Conflicting conclusions on the nature of adrenergic tonus have recently been provided by Smith (171) and by Cameron (22). In studies on the effects of bretylium and phentolamine on heart rate and dorsal aortic blood pressure in free-swimming rainbow trout, Smith concludes that systemic vascular resistance is controlled by adrenergic innervation and that increases in resistance during rapid swimming are produced by these nerves (170). The use by Wahlquist and Nilsson (189) and by Randall and Stevens (144) of the relatively nonspecific phenoxybenzamine as an α-adrenergic blocker is criticized by Smith (170). He presents different interpretations of the actions of 6-hydroxydopamine and reserpine given by Wahlquist and Nilsson (189). Smith agrees with the conclusion of Wood (196) that hemorrhage-induced oscillations of systemic vascular resistance which are eliminated by the α-adrenergic blocker yohimbine support the claim for adrenergic tonus vasomotor control in teleosts by nerves rather than circulating catecholamines. Direct measurement has recently been made of increased concentration, due to vagal nerve stimulation, of Epi, NE, and dopamine in the perfusate of isolated goldfish hearts (23). The significance of the role of sympathetic innervation in regulating fish cardiovascular systems may also vary with species and state of exercise (22).

This controversy is an excellent illustration of the need for thorough understanding of the complex actions of chemicals in fish and of the inherent responses of the basic physiological system. Additional research in each of these areas is required. For example, the mechanisms and sites of action for selective β-adrenergic vasodilation in the gill may provide insight into the regulation of dorsal aortic blood pressure in preparations similar to those used by Smith (170).

In general, pharmacological responses of the lungfish cardiovascular system resemble those seen in teleosts. Phentolamine completely blocks the pressor response by Epi and NE, and also antagonizes the increased vascular resistance produced by these catecholamines in perfusion experiments (82). A decrease in dorsal aortic blood pressure and an occasional decrease in heart rate is also seen with phentolamine, whereas propranolol produces an increase in dorsal aortic blood pressure. These observations may indicate the presence of systemic α-adrenergic receptors and branchial β-adrenergic receptors. Additional research is required, however, to understand fully the pharmacological nature of the cardiovascular responses in these animals.

The effects of phenoxybenzamine on elasmobranch circulation have been investigated in two shark species (164,165). This drug, which produces a complex triphasic response by itself, blocks the pressor response of Epi. Epi also produces a decrease in dorsal aortic blood pressure in phenoxybenzamine pretreated animals. Ergotamine and ephedrine do not alter blood pressure or affect the response of Epi in the perfused systemic vasculature of dogfish sharks (59). Neither ephedrine nor dibenamine has any effect on the heart rate or blood pressure in the intact dogfish shark circulation

(15). While the studies of Schwartz and Borzelleca (164,165) provide additional evidence for the presence of α-adrenergic and β-adrenergic receptors, the cardiovascular pharmacology of ergotamine, ephedrine, and dibenamine in these animals should be re-evaluated using technological advances of recent decades.

Evidence has been provided for the presence of α- and β-adrenergic receptors in the hagfish circulatory system (146). Perfusion of the branchial vascular bed reveals that Epi and NE produce a decrease in resistance that can be blocked by propranolol. A later increase in resistance is observed and can be blocked by phentolamine.

The early studies of McWilliam (111) demonstrating cholinergic control of the cardiovascular system in the eel have been confirmed in other teleost species (55,114,138), in elasmobranchs (103,104,105), in hagfish (146), and in lungfish (82). While results to date are equivocal, the extent of cholinergic control of the heart in resting fish may be temperature dependent (126,137).

The predominance of this cholinergic control was recently demonstrated using a novel pharmacological approach (22). In this approach, intrinsic heart rate was obtained by removing autonomic modulation with pharmacological blocking agents. Calculations demonstrated that cholinergic tone contributes 66% of autonomic control of goldfish heart rate.

A comprehensive investigation of the effects of acetylcholine (Ach) on the cardiovascular system of the Japanese eel has been presented by Chan and Chow (33). At doses less than 0.1 μg/kg, Ach produces decreases in heart rate, stroke volume, cardiac output, and in dorsal and ventral aortic mean and pulse pressures. Atropine blocks these effects, neostigmine prolongs them, and tubocurare has no influence on the Ach effects. At doses greater than 0.1 μg/kg Ach produces a biphasic response similar to, but more pronounced than, those produced at doses of less than 0.1 μg/kg. A secondary increase in arterial blood pressures is also produced, which is not affected by the ganglionic blockers hexamethonium and pentolinium, but is abolished by bretylium, phentolamine, and phenoxybenzamine. In the presence of these adrenergic antagonists, high doses of Ach still produce the decrease in heart rate and in aortic mean and pulse pressures.

In MacKay's investigations on the skate (107), Ach injected directly into the heart produced an immediate and profound decrease in heart rate. This was followed by a marked increase in ventral aortic blood pressure, which reached a maximum in 5 to 10 min and then gradually subsided. The nature and sequence of these Ach-induced effects may indicate cardiac cholinergic responses and subsequent reflex adrenergic pressor effects. Injection of Ach through the hepatic circulation markedly decreased these direct effects. Atropine abolished the cardiac effects but had only a slight effect on the pressor response.

Atropine also blocked the decrease in heart rate produced by asphyxia (116) and hypoxia (86). The magnitude of atropine's effect on bradycardia depends on the activity of the fish (79). In the dogfish shark, atropine causes a decrease in blood pressure and augments responses to other pressor agents (15). In lungfish, atropine decreases dorsal aortic blood pressure but does not alter heart rate (82). In the icefish, atropine produces slight increases in heart rate and dorsal aortic blood pressure (61).

Depressor responses, similar to those observed in the eel (33), have been produced by Ach in other species. Intraventral aortic injection of Ach in the skate produces pronounced decreases in heart rate and in dorsal and ventral aortic blood pressures (79). Intravenous administration of Ach has produced a decrease in blood pressure in the eel (113), the catfish (163), and the hemoglobin-free icefish (61).

Nicotine produces a hypotensive effect in the dogfish shark (15) and in two other shark species (164). No significant change of blood pressure is seen in the eel, even in doses of nicotine that cause generalized twitching of the body (113). In the dogfish shark, neither physostigmine nor tetraethylammonium produce an effect on blood pressure or heart rate (15), and physostigmine has no influence on the flow rate through perfused systemic vasculature (59).

*Responses to Histamine and 5-Hydroxytryptamine*

MacKay (107) commented on the variable effectiveness of histamine on the cardiovascular system of skates when she noted that "a trifling rise in blood pressure was sometimes observed" with doses greater than 10 mg per fish. Smaller doses produced a slight decrease in blood pressure, sometimes only after atropine and dihydroergokryptine were given (15,107). Although a depressor response to histamine has also been observed in the eel, it generally has very weak effects on the teleost cardiovascular system (33,113,149).

Reite (146) investigated the cardiovascular responses of two species of hagfish, five species of Chrondrichthyes, and seven species of Osteichthyes to histamine and 5-hydroxytryptamine (5-HT). In fish, 5-HT might be stored in adrenergic nerves and chromaffin cells (185). The purpose of the phylogenetic approach of Reite was to assist in elucidating the dual actions of histamine and 5-HT on vascular smooth muscle (146,147). The excitatory or inhibitory actions were viewed as separate entities and were followed not only through fish, but also into amphibia and reptiles (147,148). It was concluded that in the hagfish, histamine and 5-HT produce vascular responses that are mediated by adrenergic receptor mechanisms. Occasional and weak pressor responses to 5-HT are observed in elasmobranchs, whereas histamine does not produce any change in blood pressure. Both agonists produce specific stimulatory actions in teleost vasculature, although weak in the case of histamine. The response to both histamine and 5-HT is localized to the branchial vasculature. Histamine proves to be a rather weak agonist, whereas 5-HT produces "a powerful constriction of branchial blood vessels." A pronounced pressor response to histamine and 5-HT in the intact lungfish is also exhibited in the perfused branchial, pulmonary, and systemic vasculature of this fish (82,146).

Intravenous injection of 5-HT produces a slight decrease in dorsal aortic blood pressure in the catfish and cat shark, although "enormous doses" are needed, "e.g. 90 $\mu$g/kg for a decrease of 3 mm Hg" (163). At lower doses of 0.1 to 1.0 $\mu$g/kg in eels, 5-HT produces a decrease in heart rate that is blocked by atropine, and decreases in prebranchial and systemic blood pressures (33). In dogfish shark, 5-HT mimics the responses produced by hypoxia and hypercapnia, namely increased pregill resistance with decreased heart rate, cardiac output, and dorsal aortic blood pressure, and increased branchial resistance. Increases in ventral aortic blood pressure and decreases in heart rate are observed with lysergic acid diethylamide in the dogfish shark (194).

*Responses to Vasoactive Polypeptides*

Pressor responses to neurohypophysial peptides of mammalian origin were first observed in skates and later in eels (107,113). Extracts of fish urophysis, which is similar to mammalian neuro-hypophysis, produce an increase in blood pressure (9,32). Purified peptides of the urophysis elicit a pressor response in the eel and the lungfish (30,31,161). A dorsal aorta depressor response, which has an onset of action of 10 to 15 min and lasts for 1 to 2 hr, is reported with high doses in the eel (31).

Potency ratios for the ventral aortic pressor response in the eel were determined, assuming oxytocin to be 1.0. From this it was determined that the order of potency was: isotocin (4-Ser, 8-Ile oxytocin) 3.0; oxytocin 1.0; vasotocin (8-Arg oxytocin) 0.27; and 8-Arg vasopressin 0.007. 8-Lys vasopressin was ineffective at doses up to 20 µg/kg (31). A few investigations into the pharmacological characterization of these responses have been conducted. Atropine does not block the increase of blood pressure produced by Pitressin in the dogfish shark; however, phentolamine injected before or after the administration of isotocin abolishes the pressor response in the eel (15,30). This later observation, coupled with the very prolonged (6 to 8 hr) and tachyphylactic nature of the response, prompted an investigation into the interaction of peptides with adrenergic and cholinergic receptors (31).

In this investigation, evidence was presented favoring an adren-ergic mechanism for the ventral aortic pressor response and a cho-linergic mechanism for the depressor response in the dorsal aorta. Data presented that support the adrenergic mechanism include: (a)

NE prolongs the vasopressor response in preparations tachyphylactic to the peptides; (b) phentolamine prevents and abolishes the pressor response to isotocin; (c) a single injection of tyramine partially abolishes, while repeated injections completely abolish, the response to isotocin; and (d) cocaine augments, while bretylium antagonizes, the response to isotocin, although this is confused by the direct cardiac effects. Evidence for the cholinergic mechanism is less clear. Both atropine and tubocurarine prevented the dorsal aortic depressor response, and the authors speculate on possible cholinergic peripheral vasodilatory effects or the increased branchial resistance mechanism previously described (35).

The corpuscles of Stannius are considered to be endocrine organs associated with the kidney of holostean and teleostean fish. Although their functions are debated (9,39,62,96,185), it has been suggested that they may be functionally analogous to the renin-angiotensin system of mammals (36,173,182).

Angiotensin produces a pressor response in eels and angiotensin amide elicits a similar effect in the lungfish (32,33,36,182). Extracts of corpuscles of Stannius exert pressor responses in fish and show renin-like activity in other types of vertebrate assay systems (35,36,182). A lack of response to renin, angiotensin I, and angiotensin II has been reported in the catfish and cat shark (187). Although the investigators considered hepatic circulation, no comment was made on the possible effect of angiotensinase discussed by others (36).

Gamma-aminobutyric acid (GABA) and bradykinin in eels cause a decrease in heart rate that is prevented by atropine (33). The lack of pressor effects of bradykinin, kallikrein, kallidin, and eledoisin has been reported by Vogel et al. (187). They have observed an irreversible decrease in blood pressure produced by homogenates of fish pancreas.

## Isolated Heart Preparations

McWilliam (111) provided some of the original insight into the mechanisms of cardiovascular control in fish with his observations on the eel heart, both *in vivo* and in isolated preparations. In addition to descriptions of anatomical characteristics, the effects of nerve and direct electrical stimulation, and of vagal nerve sectioning, he commented on some pharmacological responses. The ability of "curara" to abolish the inhibitory response produced by nerve and direct stimulation was demonstrated, as well as a cardiac depressant action of strychnine which was thought to be similar to vagal stimulation.

Since McWilliam's report, additional work utilizing isolated heart preparations has assisted in providing refined techniques and knowledge of extrinsic and intrinsic cardioregulatory mechanisms (27, 38,49,50,54,55,57,65,102,106,124,138,139,155,156). In addition to these reports, which are concerned with elasmobranch and teleost fish, investigations of the peculiarities of the hearts of hagfish (50,76) and of lungfish (2,81) are available.

As previously stated, the physiological control of elasmobranch and teleost hearts is predominantly regulated by cholinergic vagal nerve fibers (24,79,114,139,156). Stimulation of these fibers and direct application of Ach produces negative inotropic and chronotropic effects in the atria that are blocked by muscarinic receptor antagonists, such as atropine (49,55,65,106,138,140). Atropine also blocks the effects of vagal stimulation and Ach application on transmembrane action potentials in atrial cells (38,155).

While the physiological significance of adrenergic innervation in fish cardiac regulation is uncertain, fish hearts, as well as other components of the cardiovascular system, are exposed to circulating catecholamines as described in the previous section. Most of the early investigators concluded that a sympathetic nerve supply to the heart was lacking (see review by Burnstock, ref. 16), but the use of electron microscopic and fluorescent histochemical techniques have demonstrated adrenergic innervation of the teleost heart (22,55,65,203). Direct evidence of catecholamine release by vagal nerve stimulation has recently been obtained in isolated, perfused goldfish hearts (23).

Pharmacological evidence favoring adrenergic neuronal control mechanisms of the isolated rainbow trout heart is provided by the investigations of Gannon and Burnstock (55) and of Gannon (54). After atropine blockade of cholinergic-induced inhibitory effects, vagal stimulation produce a cardio-excitatory response that is antagonized by the neuronal catecholamine release inhibitors bretylium and guanethidine, and by the β-adrenergic receptor blocker pronethalol. Using a field stimulation technique for selectively stimulating either adrenergic or cholinergic nerves (186), Gannon (54) studied the pharmacological responses of atria and ventricles from rainbow trout and eel. Adrenergic nerve stimulation in these atria and ventricles was blocked by the β-adrenergic receptor blocker propranolol, was potentiated by bretylium and guanethidine, and was mimicked by catecholamines in the following order of potency: Isop > Epi > NE. This study also demonstrated that atrial cholinergic nerve stimulation was blocked by atropine or hyoscine, was potentiated by the cholinesterase inhibitor neostigmine, and was mimicked by Ach and carbachol.

Other investigators have concluded that the inhibitory and excitatory responses produced by vagal stimulation are both mediated by cholinergic mechanisms. Vagal stimulation at higher frequencies produces an inhibitory response in isolated plaice hearts, whereas lower frequency stimulation produces an increase in heart rate. While bretylium and pronethalol have no effect on either response, atropine blocks both of them (38). Atropine also blocks inhibitory and excitatory responses produced by vagal stimulation in carp atria (155).

In isolated, perfused hearts from cod, vagal stimulation produced a decrease in heart rate that is blocked by atropine (65). After atropine blockade, this stimulation produces an increase in heart rate that is blocked by propranolol. In general, these perfused whole hearts are accelerated by adrenergic agonists and are depressed by Ach. Adrenergic agonist drugs produce positive inotropic effects on strips of heart and Ach has a negative inotropic effect on atrial strips. By combining these pharmacological studies with fluorescent histochemistry, Holmgren (65) concludes that in the cod the vagus supplies the heart with inhibitory cholinergic nerves and excitatory adrenergic nerves.

As described in the previous section, circulating catecholamines released from chromaffin tissue generally play a significant role in the adrenergic control of elasmobranch and teleost hearts (20, 57,65,121,157,189). Early studies demonstrated that high concentrations of Epi generally reduced heart rate in elasmobranchs (102,106). In isolated, perfused hearts of the dogfish shark, catecholamines produce positive inotropic effects in a potency order of Isop > Epi > NE (27). These effects are elicited by β-adrenergic receptors, since they are blocked by propranolol but not phentolamine. While Epi and Isop produce positive chronotropic effects, NE elicts slight negative chronotropic effects. These NE effects are mediated by α-adrenergic receptors, since they are blocked by phentolamine but are not affected by atropine or physostigmine.

Fange and Ostlund (50) concluded that the positive inotropic effects of Epi and NE are more pronounced than the positive chronotropic effects in elasmobranchs, whereas in teleosts the positive chronotropic effects predominate. Epi is approximately ten times more potent than NE in isolated teleost heart preparations (38,50,55). The effects of Epi in teleost hearts are generally mediated by β-adrenergic receptors (38,49,55,65). These receptors are the $B_2$ type in the atrium of rainbow trout (3). In isolated carp hearts, however, Epi does not elicit excitatory responses, but produces concentration-dependent inhibitory effects (155).

Other agonists have been investigated in isolated heart preparations. High concentrations of tyramine have slight positive chronotropic effects in cod and wrasse, and slight positive inotropic effects in elasmobranchs (50); positive inotropic and chronotropic effects in lamprey (49); marked positive inotropic effects in rainbow trout and eel (54); and no effects in plaice (38,49), in dogfish shark (26), or in hagfish (50). Dopamine has variable excitatory effects in cod and eel, and slight positive inotropic effects in dogfish and skate (50). Neither dopamine nor 5-HT has any effects on plaice atria (54).

## Isolated Gill Preparations

Using isolated, perfused gill preparations from pike, Krawkow (95) first reported on experiments designed to understand physiological mechanisms controlling blood flow through this unique, vital, and multifunction organ exposed directly to the aquatic environment. The entire gill apparatus was removed from the fish and the ventral aorta was cannulated and perfused under constant pressure. Vasodilatation and vasoconstriction were estimated by counting the number of drops from the cut ends of the gill arches. Epi produced a large increase in flow rate, whereas nicotine, barium chloride, and histamine produced a decrease in flow rate.

Within the last decade, many other investigations have been conducted on factors controlling branchial vascular resistance. While a couple of these investigations (87,125) have used the isolated, perfused whole gill as did Krawkow (95), many perfuse just one of the gill arches (8,10,41,64,127,145,151,152,166,170,172,190). Because of alternate routes of blood flow available in perfused head preparations (73,142,195,197,199), studies using a single arch, especially when isolated as first described by Rankin and Maetz (145), are better for evaluating sites of microcirculation control (170). Intact cardiovascular preparations with infrared photographic techniques (42), radiolabeled microspheres (21), and marking of blood cells with fluorescent dye (11) have also been used to study control mechanisms of branchial vascular resistance. A microscopic evaluation of the chemical effects on gill filaments in physiological saline on a glass slide initiated considerable controversy on the regulation of functional respiratory surface area (178).

The nonrespiratory (filamental) shunt model for control of this surface area proposed by Steen and Kruysse (178) was later supported by Richards and Fromm (151) and by Bergmann et al. (8). This model was described as having three routes of blood flow from the afferent to the efferent filamental artery, namely through secondary lamellae, a central filamental sinus (cavity), or directly from afferent to efferent artery at the tip of the filament. The route through the secondary lamellae results in respiratory gas exchange and the other two, especially the central sinus, are referred to as the non-respiratory paths (shunts). Like previous investigators (125), Richards and Fromm (151) observed that Ach and Epi predominantly produced vasoconstriction and vasodilatation, respectively, in the branchial vasculature. They suggested that Ach constricts the lamellar arterioles and directs flow to the nonrespiratory central sinus. Epi, however, was thought to cause vasodilatation of these arterioles, vasoconstriction of the central sinus vessels, and, therefore, an increase in respiratory surface area. From observations on the effects of catecholamines, adrenergic $\alpha$- and $\beta$-receptor antagonists, and Ach on $^{14}C$-urea uptake by the gills, Bergmann et al. (8) concluded that the data supported a shunt model. They also concluded that catecholamines acted on $\alpha$- and $\beta$-adrenergic receptors to increase functional surface area, and to increase or decrease branchial vascular resistance by $\alpha$- or $\beta$-adrenergic mechanisms, respectively. Stimulation of $\alpha$-adrenergic receptors was thought to produce vasoconstriction of efferent filamental arteries, which increased the blood pressure in afferent filamental arteries and caused greater perfusion of lamellar respiratory units.

In commenting on the failure of histological sections to show erythrocytes in the central sinus, of dye injections to confirm blood flow through the sinus, and of unfiltered Ringer's solution to perfuse this sinus, Hughes (68) was the first to express doubt on the validity, or at least the significance, of the nonrespiratory shunt model. Instead of shunts, Hughes (68) proposed a lamellar recruitment model to explain the regulation of blood flow. According to this model, when oxygen demand is low, blood flows only through secondary lamellae on proximal ends of filaments; when oxygen demand increases, additional lamellae toward the distal filamental tips are perfused to increase functional respiratory surface area.

In the year Hughes proposed this model, Davis (42), using an infrared photographic technique, demonstrated that intravenous injection of Epi produces an increase in branchial blood volume. While Booth (11) has described the work of Davis as direct evidence favoring lamellar recruitment, the increase in blood volume may have been due to flow shunting from a central sinus, where blood would not have been photographed, to secondary lamellae, where it was photographed.

By considering the effects of nonrespiratory shunts on oxygen saturation of dorsal aortic blood, Cameron (21) estimated that there would be less than 50% saturation if only 80% of the blood flow were oxygenated. Injection of radiolabeled microspheres in the pre-gill circulation of arctic grayling, burbot, and long-nosed suckers, subsequent histological examination and radioactivity determination were used to evaluate blood flow through a central cavity. Since microspheres were not found in a central cavity, even when Ach or Epi was injected to maximize conditions previously described for controlling blood flow shunts, Cameron (21) concluded that shunt pathways did not exist or, at most, had slight significance.

Similar conclusions have recently been made by investigators examining the distribution of Prussian Blue dye in rainbow and brown trout (170), of blood cells marked with a fluorescent dye in rainbow trout (11), and of radiolabeled erythrocytes in the channel catfish (64). Booth (11) provides an excellent summary of phys-iological studies in the nonrespiratory shunt versus lamellar recruit-ment controversy. He states that lamellar recruitment "would seem to be a better strategy for changing the functional surface area of the gills," in that it would avoid the decrease in oxygen saturation of dorsal aortic blood inherent to the shunt model, and would de-crease the work load of the heart by reducing branchial resistance during high oxygen demand periods. Additional research using blood cell marking techniques in nonstressed and stressed fish is needed to provide direct evidence of the lamellar recruitment model.

The pronounced vasodilatory response by isolated pike gills to Epi (95) was later observed in eels (87) and other teleost species (125). While Ostlund and Fange (125) were unable to demonstrate this vasodilatory response in elasmobranchs, Davies and Rankin (41) observed that Epi produced a specific, dose-related vasodila-tation in perfused dogfish shark gills. In isolated, *in situ*, perfused gills of dogfish shark, Epi and NE produces a biphasic response of vasoconstriction followed by vasodilation, whereas Isop only elicits vasodilation (28).

Investigations of catecholamines, such as NE (125,142,145), Isop (41,170,197), and phenylephrine (8,197) have been performed in other isolated, perfused gill preparations. A potency order for vasodilatation of Isop > NE > Epi with approximately equal maximal responses is observed in rainbow trout (195,197). In terms of maximum vasodilatory response, an intrinsic activity order of Epi > NE > Isop is observed in the dogfish shark (41). While phenylephrine produces an increase in vascular resistance in isolated, perfused gill arches from rainbow trout (8), Wood (195) did not observe any response in the perfused, whole gill preparation.

Adrenergic receptor antagonists have provided insight into pharmacological mechanisms mediating catecholamine-induced effects on branchial vascular resistance. Yohimbine, an α-adrenergic receptor antagonist, blocks the increased flow rate produced by Epi and NE in isolated, perfused gills of the viviparous blenny, suggesting an α-adrenergic receptor-induced vasodilatation (125). Contradictory evidence has been obtained in isolated, perfused gill arches of the eel (145). In these preparations, the increased flow rate produced by Epi and NE was blocked by the β-adrenergic antagonists propranolol, pronethalol, and dichloroisoproterenol, but not by phentolamine, an α-adrenergic antagonist. Other investigations have demonstrated both α- and β-adrenergic receptors in rainbow trout gill. In using the selective α- and β-adrenergic agonists phenylephrine and Isop, respectively, in addition to Epi and NE, and the adrenergic antagonists phenoxybenzamine, phentolamine, and propranolol, Bergmann et al. (8) concluded that stimulation of α-adrenergic receptors produces increases in functional surface area and branchial vascular resistance, whereas β-adrenergic receptor stimulation also produces an increase in functional surface area but a decrease in branchial vascular resistance. Wood (197) found that propranolol and dichloroisoproterenol blocks catecholamine-induced vasodilatation in rainbow trout and that yohimbine blocks a small constrictory response that sometimes precedes a larger dilatory effect produced by Epi and NE. Similar observations in Atlantic cod were made by Pettersson and Nilsson (127) in investigations on the effects of electrical stimulation of the nerve supply to gills on branchial vascular resistance. This stimulation produced either a decrease in vascular resistance mediated by β-adrenergic receptors or an increase in resistance that was blocked by phentolamine, leaving a decrease in resistance that was blocked by propranolol. The use of pharmacological blocking agents demonstrates that the initial vasoconstriction produced by Epi or NE in isolated, *in situ*, perfused gills of dogfish shark is mediated by α-adrenergic receptors and the vasodilatation by β-adrenergic receptors (28).

Permeability changes to water, electrolytes, and larger molecules have also been produced by catecholamines. Keys and Bateman (87) concluded that the decrease in chloride secretion produced by Epi in perfused eel gills bathed in sea water is due to either a direct inhibitory effect of Epi on chloride secretion or an increased permeability of the gills. The increase in sodium uptake produced by Epi in rainbow trout arches was shown to be "a direct stimulatory effect on the sodium-pumping mechanism (152)." The direction of sodium transport appears to be reversible, since catecholamines added to the external media bathing perfused head preparations of rainbow trout produce an increase in sodium loss across the gills (142). In the gills of salt water adapted mullet, Epi produces a decrease in net sodium extrusion rate, which is sensitive to α-adrenergic receptor blockade by phentolamine and tolazoline, but not to β-adrenergic receptor blockade by propranolol (133). Similar observations of depressed electrolyte transport mediated by an α-adrenergic mechanism were made by Shuttleworth in flounder gills (166). A β-adrenergic-mediated increase in water permeability was also produced by Epi (73,132). This water permeability effect and the increased permeability to other molecules, such as urea and butanol, are direct effects of Epi on branchial membranes and may be partially responsible for the increased oxygenation of dorsal aortic blood produced by Epi (40,72,74,128,200).

Ach-induced branchial vasoconstriction observed in elasmobranchs (41), teleosts (10,166), and the air-breathing jeju (172) is produced by muscarinic receptor mechanisms (125,127,197). The decrease in functional gill surface area and the increase in branchial resistance produced by Ach results in a decrease in the arteriovenous difference in the partial pressure of oxygen (8,40). Perfusion of isolated gill arches in orthograde or retrograde directions provides evidence that Ach acts "at a site downstream from the secondary lamellae, probably at the base of the efferent filament arteries (170)."

Other agents producing a change in branchial resistance have been investigated in a cursory fashion. Although only "a few experiments" on the viviparous blenny were conducted (125), histamine produced an increase in flow rate, instead of the vasoconstriction seen by Krawkow (95). Reite (149) stated that histamine has weak constrictory effects on branchial vasculature in most teleosts. 5-HT produces a pronounced and long-lasting vasoconstriction in the viviparous blenny (125) and a discharge in respiratory nociceptors producing reflex hypotension in the dogfish shark (136). Variable responses to Pitressin have been observed in the eel (87). The technique of visualizing gill microcirculation under a cover slip (178) has been applied to study the vasoconstrictor responses to oxytocin and vasotocin (35). These responses are also observed in isolated, perfused gill arches at extremely low concentrations, but lys-vasopressin has no effect (145).

Substantial advances in knowledge of branchial blood flow routes have been made using scanning and transmission electron microscopy (EM). The first application of scanning EM to teleost gills did not reveal central cavity shunts, but a complex microcirculatory structure that seemed to be equivalent to a nutritive capillary bed was observed (56). Complex branchial microcirculatory systems have also been photographed in the hagfish (135) and in the lamprey (118,119). Future studies related to the physiological pharmacology or toxicology of branchial microcirculation should consider the electron micrographs of Vogel (188) and of Kendall and Dale (85). These provide a truly exceptional and complimentary perspective on routes of blood flow through rainbow trout filaments (primary lamellae) and secondary lamellae.

## Isolated Vascular Preparations

As discussed in previous sections, investigations on isolated vascular preparations have dealt in large part with the pharmacological nature of adrenergic and cholinergic control mechanisms and with the significance of innervation and circulating catecholamines in adrenergic control. Since the latter aspect has been discussed to some degree in this chapter and reviews are available that deal specifically with fish cardiovascular innervation (16,157,159), this section will focus on the pharmacological nature of vascular responses.

Isolated systemic vascular responses have been investigated using three basic approaches. These are: perfused, whole, systemic vasculature (201); perfused portions, e.g., the swimbladder of the systemic vasculature (181); and isolated blood vessels, e.g., hepatic veins (80).

Adrenergic control of systemic vascular resistance in the isolated, perfused trunk of rainbow trout is largely due to $\alpha$-adrenergic vasoconstriction receptors (201). In the absence of other drugs, Epi is approximately three times more potent than NE; there are no responses to phenylephrine, methoxamine, or Isop; and dopamine and tyramine produce weak constrictive effects (198). The constrictive responses to Epi and NE were blocked by phenoxybenzamine and yohimbine and, curiously, by propranolol and dichloro-isoproterenol. Wood (198) has suggested that the effect of the $\beta$-adrenergic blocking drugs may be "due to non-competitive antagonism with a point of action beyond the adrenergic receptor." When $\alpha$-adrenergic vasoconstriction is produced, Isop elicits a vasodilatory response. Wood (198) also states that the predominance of the adrenergic vasoconstriction and the apparent lack of vasodilatation in the isolated, perfused trunk preparation "could be due to an already maximal relaxation of the resistance vessels . . . rather than to a lack of $\beta$-adrenoreceptors in the systemic vasculature."

Wood (199) has also used the isolated, perfused trunk preparation to study the mechanisms of cholinergic-induced increases in systemic vascular resistance. This increased resistance produced by

Ach has been observed in perfused vasculature of hagfish, cod, eel (146), dogfish shark (59), and lungfish (82). In rainbow trout, Ach produces a dose-dependent vasoconstriction that has two components (199). The first (component A) is a rapid and pronounced increase of short duration in perfusion pressure; the second (component B) is a long-lasting and steady increase in pressure over baseline. Component B is actually a "tail" on the component A response. Phenoxybenzamine and yohimbine decrease component B and have no effect on A; propranolol has no effect on either component; and guanethidine does not decrease A and has no effect on B. The muscarinic agonists methacholine and pilocarpine have no effects; nicotinic receptor antagonists inhibit both A and B in the following order of potency: *d*-tubocurarine gallamine > hexamethonium; atropine produces nonspecific antagonism at very high concentrations; and nicotine produces responses identical to Ach. Finally, while histamine and 5-HT have no effects, adenosine triphosphate (ATP) produces a response identical to component A. From these observations, it was concluded that response A is due either to direct stimulation of nicotine receptors in the vasculature or to release of a nonadrenergic and noncholinergic transmitter, perhaps ATP (199). Response B appears to be due to an adrenergic transmitter released by Ach action on sympathetic neurons or chromaffin tissue.

These responses to Ach have not been observed in perfused, isolated segments of the systemic vasculature or in isolated vascular preparations. In swimbladder preparations from eel (181) and cod (120), Ach produces a vasoconstriction that is blocked by atropine, indicating a muscarinic receptor-mediated mechanism. Pronounced, concentration-dependent contractions produced by Ach in isolated, helically-cut strips of ventral aorta and bulbus arteriosus from rainbow trout are blocked by atropine and methyl atropine, but not by hexamethonium or tubocurarine (90,93). Pilocarpine, a muscarinic agonist, also produces contractions that are blocked by atropine in bulbus arteriosus strips (93). While Ach produces constriction of hepatic vein lumen from skate and dogfish, antagonists are not used to characterize the receptor mechanism (80). Ach produces "weak and irregular" contractions in celiac and lienogastric arterial strips from dogfish shark (122).

An α-adrenergic vasoconstriction is produced when innervating nerves to swimbladders of eel (181) and cod (120) and to cod celiac artery (66) are electrically stimulated. This vasoconstriction is blocked by hexamethonium or mecamylamine in cod celiac artery (66), but these ganglionic blockers have no effect on cod swimbladder vasculature (120). Evidence for the presence of β-receptors mediating a vasodilatory response was obtained in eel swimbladder (181) and cod celiac artery (66), but not in cod swimbladder (120).

Although Burnstock and Kirby (18) concluded that β-adrenergic receptors were absent in teleost pregill vasculature, Klaverkamp and Dyer (93) provided indirect and direct evidence for β-adrenergic-mediated relaxations in helically-cut strips of ventral aorta from rainbow trout. In the presence of propranolol, Epi produced a 3- to 11-fold increase in contractile tension in these strips, and propranolol blocked the concentration-dependent relaxation of Ach-induced contraction produced by Isop. While Isop also produced relaxation of NE-induced contraction in strips of celiac artery from the cod, Holmgren and Nilsson (67) were unable to conclude that this vessel has β-adrenergic receptors because they did not use β-adrenergic antagonists to block the relaxation. These receptors were also present in the pregill vasculature of dogfish shark, since Isop-induced vasodilatation was blocked by propranolol, and propranolol potentiated the vasoconstriction response produced by Epi (25). Epi also produces vasodilatation in the hepatic vein of three elasmobranch species (80).

The use of isolated blood vessels has confirmed the presence of α-adrenergic receptors in the systemic vasculature of elasmobranchs and teleosts. The potencies of catecholamines in producing contractions in isolated celiac arteries from cod and rainbow trout is Epi > NE > phenylephrine (67). NE has 40% of the intrinsic activity of Epi, and dopamine has no effect in rainbow trout ventral aortic strips (93). Tyramine and amphetamine are ineffective in ventral aortic strips from brown trout and eel (89). Phentolamine blocks catecholamine-induced contractions in vessels from dogfish shark (25,122), brown trout and eel (18), cod (67), and rainbow trout (93). Other α-adrenergic antagonists used to block catechol-amine-induced vascular contractions include yohimbine (67), phen-oxybenzamine (18,67), dibenamine (18), clonidine, oxymetazoline, and xylometazoline (83).

Very little use of isolated vasculature preparations has been made to investigate other potentially vasoactive agents. Somlyo and Som-lyo (174) used helically-cut hagfish ventral and dorsal aorta to in-vestigate the responses of arginine vasopressin, oxytocin, and vasotocin. The objective of their studies was to determine if the interaction between magnesium and neurohypophysial peptides is present in the vasculature of one of the earliest vertebrates, the hagfish. Positive results were reported on the interaction of mag-nesium with the peptides, and the Somlyos speculated on the pos-sibility of hormonal control of branchial circulation. Histamine and 5-HT had no effects in the perfused trunk preparation of Wood (199), whereas 5-HT had pronounced vasoconstriction effects in isolated pregill vasculature (92). Investigations on angiotensins in perfused vasculature of isolated dogfish gut have provided under-standing about the mode and site of action of the pressor effect of angiotensins in intact elasmobranch vasculature (123).

## THE PHYSIOLOGICAL TOXICOLOGY OF FISH CARDIOVASCULAR SYSTEMS

The investigations reviewed in the previous section on physio-logical pharmacology generally have a comparative approach for understanding evolutionary processes as one of their major objec-tives. A few of the earlier researchers, however, realized the sig-nificance of their work for the protection of fish from environmental pollution. For example, in 1930, Lutz (103) suggested that vagal inhibition of fish heart function "would serve to decrease absorption of toxic substances by the gills."

In general, the use of fish physiological responses in aquatic toxicology research programs is less than a decade old. In com-menting on attempts to relate physiological toxicology to chronic toxicity studies in 1973, Eaton (48) stated that "for the most part, investigations in these areas (physiological toxicology) are just beginning, and results are not yet available." As recently as 1977, about the common chemical element zinc, Hughes and Adeney (70) stated that few investigations "have emphasized the truly physiological approach by monitoring physiological parameters when fish were subjected to lethal concentrations of heavy metals."

The use of physiological responses in fish toxicology studies generally emphasizes one of three major objectives. The first, a category defined as "acute, sublethal toxicity tests," attempts to use these responses as sensitive and rapid tests for estimating potential adverse environmental effects of chemicals in water. The second, defined as true "bioassays," uses these responses to indicate the presence and relative quantity of a chemical or group of chemicals in solution. The third, referred to as "mechanism of action studies," investigates how chemicals produce adverse effects, generally death, in fish.

Comparisons between laboratories, species, and water quality are very difficult since the use of a single fish species and reference chemical to develop acute, sublethal toxicity tests, including cardiovascular responses, generally does not occur in one laboratory. In our laboratory, fenitrothion has been evaluated on rainbow trout using several acute, sublethal toxicity tests (Table 1). As a cholinesterase inhibitor, this organophosphate insecticide may be expected to produce effects on the cholinergically innervated cardiovascular system of fish (63,94). Table 1, however, shows that concentrations producing death in fingerlings were required to alter heart rate in adult rainbow trout. The most sensitive responses in this series of toxicity tests were cholinesterase inhibition in brain and skeletal muscle of fingerlings (juveniles) and increased cough frequency in adults.

The coughing reflex of fish, first proposed as a toxicity test response by Belding (7), consists of an abrupt reversal of water flow direction across the gills and is thought to be a response to irritation or some other form of mechanical stimulation (69). While the physiological significance of coughing is not known, it probably

TABLE 1. *A summary of responses of four life history stages of rainbow trout to fenitrothion*

| Life stage | Fenitrothion concentration, mg/liter | Exposure duration, hr | Response |
|---|---|---|---|
| Embryo | | | |
| age: 3 days before hatch | 34 | 24 | No mortality; 76% ChE inhibition |
| Sac fry | | | |
| age: 0 to 5 days | 34 | 24 | No mortality; 78% ChE inhibition at day = 0 |
| age: 6 to 9 days | 34 | 24 | Partial mortality; 84% ChE inhibition in survivors at day = 8 |
| age: 10 to 11 days | 34 | 24 | 100% mortality |
| Fingerling | 0.75 to 10.0 | 24 | $LC_{50}$ = 3.4 mg/liter |
| | | 96 | $LC_{50}$ = 2.0 mg/liter |
| | 0.75 | 96 | 75% brain ChE inhibition |
| | | 96 | 49% skeletal muscle ChE inhibition |
| Adult | 5 | 24 | Decreased heart rate |
| | 5 | 24 | increased ventilation rate |
| | 0.5 | 24 | increased cough frequency |

From Klaverkamp et al. (91).

TABLE 2. *Effects of selected chemicals in an acute sublethal toxicity test[a] for cardiovascular and respiratory functions in rainbow trout*

| Chemical | $LC_{50}$[b] (mg/l) | H.R.[c] $(l/LC_{50})$ | V.R.[d] $(l/LC_{50})$ | C.F.[e] $(l/LC_{50})$ | B.A.[f] $(l/LC_{50})$ |
|---|---|---|---|---|---|
| Acephate | 2,890 | .69 ↓ | .69 ↑ | NE | .69 ↑ |
| Acetone | 6,100 | NE | .48 ↑ | NE | .48 ↑ |
| Copper | .26 | NE | NE | .81 ↑ | NE |
| Ethanol | 11,200 | NE | .26 ↑ | NE | NE |
| Fenitrothion | 3.4 | .74 ↓ | .74 ↑ | .15 ↑ | .74 ↑ |
| Propylene glycol | > 50,000 | slight ↑ | slight ↑ | NE | NE |
| Vanadium | 35.0 | NE | .36 ↑ | .71 ↑ | NE |

[a]Procedures described in Majewski et al. (110).

[b]$LC_{50}$ = Lethal concentration for 50% of the population; with the exception of vanadium which is the 40 hr value, all values are obtained after 24 hr exposure.

[c]H.R. = Heart rate. Concentration is expressed as the fraction of the $LC_{50}$ concentration producing a change in response. Direction of change is indicated by arrow.

[d]V.R. = Ventilation rate. Concentrations and direction of change are expressed as in Heart Rate.

[e]C.F. = Cough frequency. Concentrations and direction of change are expressed as in Heart Rate.

[f]B.A. = Buccal pressure amplitude. Concentrations and direction of change are expressed as in Heart Rate.

N.E. = No effect.

Acephate and fenitrothion are organophosphate insecticides.

reduces oxygen uptake by interfering with normal countercurrent exchange mechanisms (43). Cough rate has been measured by observing pressure changes in cannulated buccal and opercular cavities of large fish (160) or only in the buccal cavity of small fish (162), by direct observation with a stopwatch (167), and, in free-swimming fish, by unimplanted electrodes (46,154,176,179). Increased cough frequency has been used as a sensitive indicator of single chemicals, such as chlorine (6), copper (46), 1,1,1,-trichloro,2,2,-bis (4-chlorophenyl) ethane (DDT) (101,162), dieldrin (101), fenitrothion (13), mercury, methyl mercury (45), zinc (69,167,175), and of complex mixtures in whole industrial effluents (5,43,69,84,191). Researchers interested in using fish respiratory

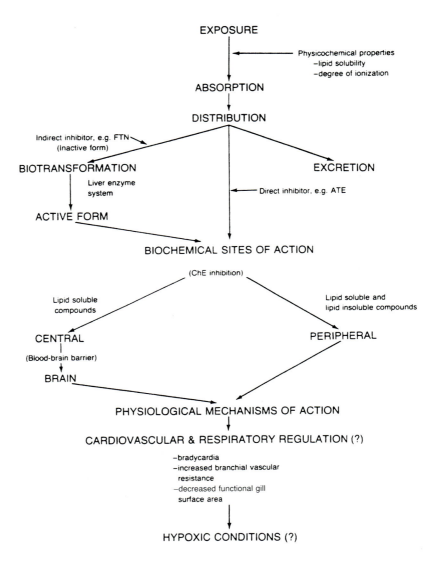

**FIG. 2.** A synopsis of the fundamental pharmacological and toxicological factors affecting acephate (ATE) and fenitrothion (FTN) toxicity to rainbow trout. (From Duangsawadi and Klaverkamp, ref. 47.)

responses as acute, sublethal toxicity tests for a large variety of chemicals are referred to the recent presentations of Carlson and Drummond (29) and of Slooff (168).

Electrocardiogram (ECG) recordings, because of the relative ease of obtaining them, are the most common measurement of cardiovascular function used as toxicity tests. These recordings, expressed in terms of heart rate and waveform changes, have been obtained using implanted pins (4), fish hooks (101), commercially available ECG electrodes (91,110), and unimplanted electrodes (154,179,180). Decreases in heart rate have been produced by low dissolved oxygen, cyanide (4), DDT, dieldrin (101), zinc (70,167), chlorine (6), phthalate esters (130), organophosphate insecticides (91), and oil spill dispersants (88). Increases in heart rate have been produced by tricaine methanesulfonate (MS222), quinaldine, urethane (99), phosphate (180), ammonia (169), cadmium (109), and an oil spill dispersant (84). Asphyxiation and cyanide produce an increase in the P-R interval and a reduction in the amplitude of the QRS complex (4). While ethanol has no effect on heart rate, there is a significant decrease in the Q-T interval with it (110). Table 2 summarizes results obtained in our laboratory using an acute, sublethal toxicity test described by Majewski et al. (110) for cardiovascular and respiratory functions of rainbow trout.

Confusion in meaning and use between the terms "bioassay" and "toxicity test" still remains in spite of frequent attempts to clarify these two concepts. A toxicity test, as can be seen from the preceding, is conducted to determine the adverse effects of chemicals contaminating water and producing a reduction in the quality of water for aquatic organisms (12). The term "bioassay" is largely associated with the measurement of concentrations of drugs, frequently of biological origin, by the determination of the strength of a stimulus by the response magnitude of a biological system.

Fish cardiovascular systems have recently been used as true bioassays in a unique set of experiments originally designed to study fish crowding factors (53). These factors, which can be extracted from water using charcoal or organic solvents, are substances released by crowded fish that prevent spawning and hatching of eggs, decrease growth, and increase mortality. By direct observation of beating hearts in newly hatched goldfish fry and by ECG recordings obtained from juvenile fish, Francis et al. (53) found excellent correlation between the decreases in average weight gain and heart rate produced by increases in fish density. The effects on heart rate are species-specific and reversed by atropine. Biochemical techniques for isolating the biologically active fraction of crowding factors revealed that these fish were also contaminated with phthalic acid esters (131). Two of these esters, especially di-*n*-butyl phthalate, were found to have substantial cardiodepressor activity (129,130).

Investigations designed to help understand the mechanism of action of chemicals with adverse effects on fish comprise the third category of physiological toxicology studies using cardiovascular responses. These studies generally expand the techniques employed in "toxicity test" and "bioassay" studies to include measurements of blood gases, pH, electrolytes, and pressures, as well as physiological respiratory responses.

Rainbow trout exposed to lethal concentrations of zinc exhibit cardiovascular and respiratory responses similar to hypoxic fish (143,167,183). In zinc-exposed fish, decreases in oxygen partial pressure in dorsal aortic blood, in oxygen utilization, and in heart rate were observed along with increases in gill ventilation volume and cough rate (167). Skidmore (167) stated that "the bradycardia in [these] zinc-poisoned fish is believed to be the first report of the phenomenon in a fish uninfluenced by drugs and with a high concentration of accessible oxygen in the surrounding environment." He concluded that the mechanism of action of zinc-induced death was tissue hypoxia caused by insufficient oxygen supply even in the presence of maximum gill ventilation. Investigations at the biochemical level have supported this conclusion (19). In extending the work of Skidmore (167), Hughes and Adeney (70) observed that zinc produced an increase in coupling between cardiovascular and respiratory rhythms. While they thought their results were influenced by the very high cough rate produced by elevated ammonia build-up in their closed system, Hughes and Adeney concluded that zinc interfered with oxygen uptake mechanisms of the gills.

Ammonia, however, does not affect cough rate in rainbow trout (169). Lethal concentrations produced substantial increases in ventilation volume, frequency and amplitude, and in heart rate, dorsal aortic blood pressure, and cardiac output, but there were no changes in cough frequency, erythrocyte number, hematocrit, hemoglobin concentration, and blood pH. The partial pressure of oxygen in dorsal aortic blood decreased to approximately 44% of control, and half the exposed fish were in a comatose state. From these observations, Smart (169) suggests that the mechanism of lethal action in fish is the same as in mammals, which is an impairment on cerebral energy metabolism.

The fish anesthetics MS222, quinaldine and urethane, produce a two-phase response in heart rate of rainbow trout (99). An initial rapid increase in heart rate (phase 1) is followed by a prolonged decrease in heart rate (phase 2). By injecting Ach, Epi, and pharmacological antagonists in the presence of anesthetic exposure, it was concluded that phase 1 was due to stress-induced catecholamine release and that phase 2 was a reflex bradycardia due to hypoxia produced by anesthetic-induced respiratory depression.

Lethal concentrations of chlorine also appear to produce reflex bradycardia due to hypoxia (6). A chlorine-induced, 15-fold increase in cough rate, which precedes an increase in ventilation frequency, may have been responsible for the 60% reduction in oxygen partial pressure of dorsal aortic blood. A subsequent shift to some anerobic metabolism is indicated by increased blood lactate and decreased blood pH. Bass and Heath (6) concluded that "free chlorine kills fish by internal hypoxia induced by damage to the gills."

Organophosphate insecticides, such as acephate and fenitrothion, may also cause death in fish by producing hypoxia (47). Guided by knowledge of sites and mechanisms of action of organophosphate insecticides in mammals, Duangsawasdi and Klaverkamp (47) attempted to understand the mechanism of the acute, lethal action of these chemicals in fish by relating brain and skeletal muscle cholinesterase inhibition to physiological parameters, such as heart, ventilation, and cough rates, and respiratory amplitude, and to cholinesterase inhibition of other organs and tissues, such as erythrocytes, gill, heart, and serum. By evaluating the time course and magnitude of effects, they suggested that these chemicals produce death by causing hypoxia. The mechanism, however, was thought to involve direct effects on the gills, rather than central nervous system and skeletal muscle (diaphragm) mechanisms producing respiratory paralysis in mammals. Figure 2 presents a synopsis of the fundamental pharmacological and toxicological factors that may affect organophosphate toxicity to fish. Many of these factors may also apply to other classes of chemicals.

Cadmium, at approximately 40% of the incipient lethal concentration, produced hypoxia in rainbow trout during chronic exposure experiments (109). Slight, but significant, increases in cardiac and ventilatory rates, hematocrit, and hemoglobin were observed during the entire exposure period, while erythrocyte ATP concentrations decreased in the later stages of exposure. Decreased oxygen saturation of hemoglobin was caused in part by a reduction in oxygen affinity of hemoglobin. Cadmium also produced a reduction in branchial oxygen transfer since decreased dorsal aortic oxygen content was observed during increased ventilation rate and buccal pressure amplitude.

Hypoxia caused by interference of gill respiratory mechanisms may be a common toxicological mechanism for many classes of chemicals. Examples of branchial mechanisms that could result in hypoxia include increased coughing frequency, increased mucus formation, depression of aerobic metabolic processes, vasoconstriction in secondary lamellae, skeletal muscle paralysis, and loss of oxygen sensory ability. These and other mechanisms could result in hypoxia much more readily in fish than in air-breathing vertebrates, since there is a much smaller quantity (approximately 3% at 15°C) of oxygen contained within a given mass of water than in an equal mass of air (158).

In conclusion, of the three categories of fish cardiovascular physiology studies directed toward toxicological objectives, those concerned with understanding the mechanisms by which chemicals produce adverse effects are likely to be the most valuable. Since powerful homeostatic mechanisms regulate cardiovascular function within relatively narrow limits, the use of cardiovascular responses, such as heart rate, as "toxicity tests" are generally not very "sensitive." The use of these responses as "bioassays" for quantifying chemical stimuli will probably continue to be limited in use as they are very stimulus-specific. Investigations to obtain knowledge on the physiological mechanisms of toxic action of chemicals in fish, however, are sorely needed. This knowledge, especially when combined with studies on biochemical and histological effects, is urgently required to direct field monitoring programs designed to detect chemical pollution of natural waters.

## ACKNOWLEDGMENTS

I am very grateful for the excellent assistance and cooperation given by Adele Yakimischak in obtaining copies of many references from various libraries and in typing all drafts of this chapter. The constructive reviews of research colleagues M. A. Giles, H. S. Majewski, and E. Scherer at the Freshwater Institute, of J. L. Hedtke at the University of Oregon Health Sciences Center in Portland, Oregon, and of G. H. Satchell at Otago University in Dunedin, New Zealand greatly improved the quality of the manuscript.

## REFERENCES

1. Albers, C. (1970): Acid-Base Balance. In: *Fish Physiology*, Vol. IV., edited by W. S. Hoar and D. J. Randall, pp. 173–208. Academic Press, New York.
2. Anthonioz, P. P., Mohsen, T., and Jadoun, G. (1978): Preuves histochimiques et ultrastructurales de l'innervation du coeur de *Protopterus annectens* (Poisson Dipneuste). *C. R. Soc. Biol.*, 172:208–211.
3. Ask, J. A., Stene-Larsen, G., and Helle, K. B. (1980): Atrial B$_2$-adrenoreceptors in the trout. *J. Comp. Physiol.*, 139:109–115.
4. Bahr, T. G. (1973): Electrophysiological responses of trout to dissolved oxygen and cyanide. In: *Bioassay Techniques and Environmental Chemistry*, edited by G. E. Glass, pp. 231–255. Ann Arbor Science Publishers, Inc., Ann Arbor, Michigan.
5. Barnett, J., and Toews, D. (1978): The effects of crude oil and the dispersant, Oilsperse 43, on respiration and coughing rates in Atlantic salmon (*Salmo salar*). *Can. J. Zool.*, 56:307–310.

6. Bass, M. L., and Heath, A. G. (1977): Cardiovascular and respiratory changes in rainbow trout (*Salmo gairdneri*) exposed intermittently to chlorine. *Water Res.*, 11:497–502.
7. Belding, D. L. (1929): The respiratory movements of fish as an indicator of a toxic environment. *Trans. Am. Fish. Soc.*, 59:239–245.
8. Bergman, H. L., Olson, K. R., and Fromm, P. O. (1974): The effects of vasoactive agents on the functional surface area of isolated-perfused gills of rainbow trout. *J. Comp. Physiol.*, 94:267–286.
9. Bern, H. A. (1967): Hormones and endocrine glands of fishes. *Science*, 158:455–462.
10. Bolis, L., and Rankin, J. C. (1978): Vascular effects of acetylcholine, catecholamines, and detergents on isolated perfused gills of pink salmon, (*Oncorhynchus gorbuscha*), coho salmon (*O. Kisutch*), and chum salmon, (*O. Keta*). *J. Fish Biol.*, 13:543–547.
11. Booth, J. H. (1978): The distribution of blood flow in the gills of fish: Application of a new technique to rainbow trout (*Salmo gairdneri*). *J. Exp. Biol.*, 73:119–129.
12. Brown, V. M. (1973): Concepts and outlook in testing the toxicity of substances to fish. In: *Bioassay Techniques and Environmental Chemistry*, edited by G. E. Glass, pp. 73–95. Ann Arbor Science Publishers, Inc., Ann Arbor, Michigan.
13. Bull, C. J., and McInerney, J. E. (1974): Behavior of juvenile coho salmon (*Oncorhynchus kisutch*) exposed to Sumithion (Fenitrothion), an organophosphate insecticide. *J. Fish Res. Board Can.*, 31:1,867–1,872.
14. Bunge, R., Johnson, M., and Ross, C. D. (1978): Nature and nurture in development of the autonomic neuron. *Science*, 199:1,409–1,416.
15. Burger, J. W., and Bradley, S. E. (1951): The general form of circulation in the dogfish, *Squalus acanthias*. *J. Cell. Comp. Physiol.*, 37:389–401.
16. Burnstock, G. (1969): Evolution of the autonomic innervation of visceral and cardiovascular systems in vertebrates. *Pharmacol. Rev.*, 21:247–324.
17. Burnstock, G. (1978): Do some sympathetic neurones synthesize and release both noradrenaline and acetylcholine? *Prog. Neurobiol.*, 11:205–222.
18. Burnstock, G., and Kirby, S. (1968): Absence of inhibitory effects of catecholamines on lower vertebrate arterial strip preparations. *J. Pharm. Pharmacol.*, 20:404–406.
19. Burton, D. T., Jones, A. J., and Cairns, Jr., J. (1972): Acute zinc toxicity to rainbow trout (*Salmo gairdneri*): Confirmation of the hypothesis that death is related to tissue hypoxia. *J. Fish Res. Board Can.*, 29:1,463–1,466.
20. Butler, P. J., Taylor, E. W., Capra, M. F., and Davison, W. (1978): The effect of hypoxia on the levels of circulating catecholamines in the dogfish *Scyliorhinus canicula*. *J. Comp. Physiol.*, 127:325–330.
21. Cameron, J. S. (1974): Evidence for the lack of by-pass shunting in teleost gills. *J. Fish Res. Board Can.*, 31:211–213.
22. Cameron, J. S. (1979): Autonomic nervous tone and regulation of heart rate in the goldfish, *Carassius auratus*. *Comp. Biochem. Physiol.*, 63C:341–349.

23. Cameron, J. S., and O'Connor, E. F. (1979): Liquid chromatographic demonstration of catecholamine release in fish heart. *J. Exp. Zool.*, 209:473–479.

24. Campbell, G. (1970): Autonomic nervous systems. In: *Fish Physiology*, vol. IV, edited by W. S. Hoar and D. J. Randall, pp. 109–132. Academic Press, New York.

25. Capra, M. F., and Satchell, G. H. (1974): Beta-adrenergic dilatory responses in isolated saline perfused arteries of an elasmobranch fish, *Squalus acanthias. Experientia*, 30:927–928.

26. Capra, M. F., and Satchell, G. H. (1977a): The differential haemodynamic responses of the elasmobranch, *Squalus acanthias*, to the naturally occurring catecholamines adrenaline and noradrenaline. *Comp. Biochem. Physiol.*, 58C:41–47.

27. Capra, M. F., and Satchell, G. H. (1977b): Adrenergic and cholinergic responses of the isolated, saline-perfused heart of the elasmobranch fish *Squalus acanthias. Gen. Pharmacol.*, 8:59–65.

28. Capra, M. F., and Satchell, G. H. (1977c): The adrenergic responses of isolated, saline-perfused prebranchial arteries and gills of the elasmobranch *Squalus acanthias. Gen. Pharmacol.*, 8:67–71.

29. Carlson, R. W., and Drummond, R. A. (1978): Fish cough response—A method for evaluating quality of treated complex effluents. *Water Res.*, 12:1–6.

30. Chan, D. K. O., and Chester Jones, I. (1967): The regulation of blood pressure in the european eel *Anguilla anguilla L.* (Abstract). *Gen. Comp. Endocrinol.*, 9:439.

31. Chan, D. K. O., and Chester Jones, I. (1969): Pressor effects of neurohypophysial peptides in the eel, *Anguilla anguilla L.*, with some reference to their interaction with adrenergic and cholinergic receptors. *J. Endocrinol.*, 45:161–174.

32. Chan, D. K. O., Chester Jones, I., and Ponniah, S. (1969): Studies on the pressor substances of the caudal neurosecretory system of teleost fish: Bioassay and fractionation. *J. Endocrinol.*, 45:151–159.

33. Chan, D. K. O., and Chow, P. H. (1976): The effects of acetylcholine, biogenic amines, and other vasoactive agents on the cardiovascular functions of the eel *Anguilla japonica. J. Exp. Zool.*, 196:13–26.

34. Chester Jones, I., Chan, D. K. O., and Rankin, J. C. (1969): Renal function in the european eel (*Anguilla anguilla L.*): Changes in blood pressure and renal function of the freshwater eel transferred to sea water. *J. Endocrinol.*, 43:9–19.

35. Chester Jones, I., Henderson, I. W., Chan, D. K. O., and Rankin, J. C. (1967): Steroids and pressor substances in bony fish with special reference to the adrenal cortex and corpuscles of stannius in the eel (*Anguilla anguilla L.*). Proc. Second International Congress on Hormonal Steroids, edited by L. Martini, F. Fraschini. and M. Motta. *International Congress Series*, 132:136–145.

36. Chester Jones, I., Henderson, I. W., Chan, D. K. O., Rankin, J. C., Mosley, W., Brown, J. J., Lever, A. F., Robertson, J. I. S., and Tree, M. (1966): Pressor activity in extracts of the corpuscles of stannius from the european eel (*Anguilla anguilla L.*). *J. Endocrinol.*, 34:393–408.

37. Chow, P. H., and Chan, D. K. O. (1975): The cardiac cycle and the effects of neurohumors on myocardial contractility in the asiatic eel *Anguilla japonica*, Timm. and Schle. *Comp. Biochem. Physiol.*, 52C:41–45.

38. Cobb, J. L. S., and Santer, R. M. (1973): Electrophysiology of cardiac function in teleosts: Cholinergically mediated inhibited and rebound excitation. *J. Physiol.*, 230:561–573.

39. Colombo, L., Bern, H. A., and Peprzyk, J. (1971): Steroid transformations by the corpuscles of stannius and the body kidney of *Salmo gairdnerii* (*Teleostei*). *Gen. Comp. Endocrinol.*, 16:74–84.

40. D'Amico Martel, A. L., and Cech, Jr., J. J. (1978): Peripheral vascular resistance in the gills of the winter flounder *Pseudopleuronectes americanus*. *Comp. Biochem. Physiol.*, 59A:419–423.

41. Davies, D. T., and Rankin, J. C. (1973): Adrenergic receptors and vascular responses to catecholamines of perfused dogfish gills. *Comp. Gen. Pharmacol.*, 4:139–147.

42. Davis, J. C. (1972): An infrared photographic technique useful for studying vascularization of fish gills. *J. Fish Res. Board Can.*, 29:109–111.

43. Davis, J. C. (1973): Sublethal effects of bleached kraft pulp mill effluent on respiration and circulation in sockeye salmon (*Oncorhynchus nerka*). *J. Fish Res. Board Can.*, 30:369–377.

44. Dornesco, G. T., and Santa, V. (1963): La structure des aortes et des vaisseaux sanguins de la carpe (*Cyprinus carpio L.*). *Anat. Anz.*, 113:136–145.

45. Drummond, R. A., Olson, G. F., and Batterman, A. R. (1974): Cough response and uptake of mercury by brook trout, *Salvelinus fontinalis*, exposed to mercuric compounds at different hydrogen ion concentrations. *Trans. Am. Fish Soc.*,103:244–249.

46. Drummond, R. A., Spoor, W. A., and Olson, G. F. (1973): Some short-term indicators of sublethal effects of copper on brook trout, *Salvelinus fontinalis*. *J. Fish Res. Board Can.*, 30:698–701.

47. Duangsawasdi, M., and Klaverkamp, J. F. (1979): Acephate and fenitrothion toxicity in rainbow trout: Effects of temperature stress and investigations on the sites of action. In: *Aquatic Toxicology*, ASTM STP 667, edited by L. L. Marking and R. A. Kimerle, pp. 35–51. American Society for Testing and Materials, Philadelphia.

48. Eaton, J. G. (1973): Recent developments in the use of laboratory bioassays to determine "safe" levels of toxicants for fish. In: *Bioassay Techniques and Environmental Chemistry*, edited by G. E. Glass, pp. 107–115. Ann Arbor Science Publishers, Inc. Ann Arbor, Michigan.

49. Falck, B., Mechklenbury, C. V., Myhrberg, H., and Persson, H. (1966): Studies on adrenergic and cholinergic receptors in the isolated hearts of *Lampetra*

*fluviatilis* (Cyclostomata) and *Pleuronectes platessa* (Teleostei). *Acta Physiol. Scand.*, 68:64–71.

50. Fange, R., and Ostlund, E. (1954): The effects of adrenaline, noradrenaline, tyramine, and other drugs on the isolated heart from marine vertebrates and a cephalopod (*Eledone cirrosa*). *Acta Zool.*, 35:289–305.

51. Forster, M. E. (1976*a*): Effects of catecholamines on the heart and on branchial and peripheral resistances of the eel *Anguilla anguilla. Comp. Biochem. Physiol.*, 55C:27–32.

52. Forster, M. E. (1976*b*): Effects of adrenergic blocking drugs on the cardiovascular system of the eel *Anguilla anguilla* (L). *Comp. Biochem. Physiol.*, 55C:33–36.

53. Francis, A. A., Smith, F., and Pfuderer, P. (1974): A heart-rate bioassay for crowding factors in goldfish. *Prog. Fish Cult.*, 36:196–200.

54. Gannon, B. J. (1971): A study of the dual innervation of teleost heart by a field stimulation technique. *Comp. Gen. Pharmacol.*, 2:175–183.

55. Gannon, B. J., and Burnstock, G. (1969): Excitatory adrenergic innervation of the fish heart. *Comp. Biochem. Physiol.*, 29:765–773.

56. Gannon, B. J., Campbell, G., and Randall, D. J. (1973): Scanning electron microscopy of vascular casts for the study of vessel connections in a complex vascular bed—The trout gill. *Proc. E. M. Soc. Am.*, 31:442–443.

57. Gannon, B. J., Campbell, G. D., and Satchell, G. H. (1972): Monoamine storage in relation to cardiac regulation in the Port Jackson Shark *Heterodontus portusjacksoni. Z. Zellforsch.*, 131:437–450.

58. Garey, W. (1970): Cardiac output of the carp (*Cyprinus carpio*). *Comp. Biochem. Physiol.*, 33:181–189.

59. Halsey, J. T., and Minnich, B. (1938): A study of the action of certain drugs on the vessels of the dogfish. *Bull. Mt. Desert Island Biol. Lab.* (40th session), 1938:16–18.

60. Hart, J. S. (1943): The cardiac output of four freshwater fish. *Can. J. Res.*, 21:77–84.

61. Hemmingsen, E. A., Douglas, E. L., Johansen, K., and Millard, R. W. (1972): Aortic blood flow and cardiac output in the hemoglobin-free fish *Chaenocephalus aceratus. Comp. Biochem. Physiol.*, 43A:1,045–1,051.

62. Heyl, H. L. (1970): Changes in the corpuscle of Stannius during the spawning journey of Atlantic salmon. *Gen. Comp. Endocrinol.*, 14:43–52.

63. Hobden, B. R., and Klaverkamp, J. F. (1977): A pharmacological characterization of acetylcholinesterase from rainbow trout (*Salmo gairdneri*) brain. *Comp. Biochem. Physiol.*, 57C:131–133.

64. Holbert, P. W., Boland, E. J., and Olson, K. R. (1979): The effect of epinephrine and acetylcholine on the distribution of red cells within the gills of the channel catfish (*Ictalurus punctatus*). *J. Exp. Biol.*, 79:135–146.

65. Holmgren, S. (1977): Regulation of the heart of a teleost, *Gadus morhua*, by autonomic nerves and circulating catecholamines. *Acta Physiol. Scand.*, 99:62–74.

66. Holmgren, S. (1978): Sympathetic innervation of the coeliac artery from a teleost, *Gadus morhua*. *Comp. Biochem. Physiol.*, 60C:27–32.

67. Holmgren, S., and Nilsson, S. (1974): Drug effects on isolated artery strips from two teleosts, *Gadus morhua* and *Salmo gairdneri*. *Acta Physiol. Scand.*, 90:431–437.

68. Hughes, G. M. (1972): Morphometrics of fish gills. *Respir. Physiol.*, 14:1–25.

69. Hughes, G. M. (1975): Coughing in the rainbow trout (*Salmo gairdneri*) and the influence of pollutants. *Rev. Suisse Zool.*, 82:47–64.

70. Hughes, G. M., and Adeney, R. J. (1977): The effects of zinc on the cardiac and ventilatory rhythms of rainbow trout (*Salmo gairdneri*, Richardson) and their responses to environmental hypoxia. *Water Res.*, 11:1,069–1,077.

71. Irisawa, H. (1978): Comparative physiology of the cardiac pacemaker mechanism. *Physiol. Rev.*, 58:461–498.

72. Isaia, J. (1979): Nonelectrolyte permeability of trout gills: Effect of temperature and adrenaline. *J. Physiol.*, 286:361–373.

73. Isaia, J., Girard, J. P., and Payan, P. (1978a): Kinetic study of gill epithelium permeability to water diffusion in the freshwater trout (*Salmo gairdneri*): Effect of adrenaline. *J. Membr. Biol.*, 41:337–347.

74. Isaia, J., Maetz, J., and Haywood, G. P. (1978b): Effects of epinephrine on branchial nonelectrolyte permeability in rainbow trout. *J. Exp. Biol.*, 74:227–237.

75. Itazawa, Y. (1970): Heart rate, cardiac output, and circulation time of fish. *Bull. Jap. Soc. Sci. Fisheries*, 36:926–932.

76. Jensen, D. (1965): The aneural heart of the hagfish. *Ann. N. Y. Acad. Sci.*, 127:443–458.

77. Johansen, K. (1962): Cardiac output and pulsatile aortic flow in the teleost, *Gadus morhua*. *Comp. Biochem. Physiol.*, 7:169–174.

78. Johansen, K. (1971): Comparative physiology: Gas exchange and circulation in fishes. *Ann. Rev. Physiol.*, 33:569–612.

79. Johansen, K., Franklin, D. L., and Van Citters, R. L. (1966): Aortic blood flow in free-swimming elasmobranchs. *Comp. Biochem. Physiol.*, 19:151–160.

80. Johansen, K., and Hanson, D. (1967): Hepatic vein sphincters in elasmobranchs and their significance in controlling hepatic blood flow. *J. Exp. Biol.*, 46:195–203.

81. Johansen, K., and Hanson, D. (1968): Functional anatomy of the hearts of lungfishes and amphibians. *Am. Zool.*, 8:191–210.

82. Johansen, K., and Reite, O. B. (1968): Influence of acetylcholine and biogenic amines on branchial, pulmonary, and systemic vascular resistance in the african lungfish *Protopterus aethiopicus*. *Acta Physiol. Scand.*, 74:465–471.

83. Johansson, P. (1979): Antagonistic effects of synthetic alpha-adrenoceptor agonists on isolated artery strips from the cod *Gadus morhua*. *Comp. Biochem. Physiol.*, 63C:267–268.

84. Johnstone, A. D. F., and Hawkins, A. D. (1980): Changes in the respiration and blood circulation of cod, *Gadus morhua*, induced by exposure to pollutants. Department of Agriculture and Fisheries for Scotland, Marine Laboratory, 40 p. (Scottish fisheries research project; no. 18 ISSN 0308–8022), Aberdeen.

85. Kendall, M. W., and Dale, J. E. (1979): Scanning and transmission electron microscopic observations of rainbow trout (*Salmo gairdneri*) gill. *J. Fish Res. Board Can.*, 36:1,072–1,079.

86. Kent, B., and Pierce, III, E. C. (1978): Cardiovascular responses to changes in blood gases in dogfish shark, *Squalus acanthias*. *Comp. Biochem. Physiol.*, 60C:37–44.

87. Keys, A., and Bateman, J. B. (1932): Branchial responses to adrenaline and to pitressin in the eel. *Biol. Bull.*, 63:327–336.

88. Kiceniuk, J. W., Penrose, W. R., and Squires, W. R. (1978): Oil spill dispersants cause bradycardia in a marine fish. *Marine Poll. Bull.*, 9:42–45.

89. Kirby, S., and Burnstock, G. (1969): Comparative pharmacology studies of isolated spiral strips of large arteries from lower vertebrates. *Comp. Biochem. Physiol.*, 28:307–319.

90. Klaverkamp, J. F. (1975): Effects of pH on cholinergic vascular receptors of rainbow trout *Salmo gairdneri*. *Gen. Pharmacol.*, 6:9–14.

91. Klaverkamp, J. F., Duangsawasdi, M., Macdonald, W. A., and Majewski, H. S. (1977): An evaluation of fenitrothion toxicity in four life stages of rainbow trout *Salmo gairdneri*. In: *Aquatic Toxicology and Hazard Evaluation*, ASTM STP 634, edited by F. L. Mayer and J. L. Hamelink, pp. 231–240. American Society for Testing and Materials, Philadelphia.

92. Klaverkamp, J. F., and Dyer, D. C. (1971): Cholinergic and serotonergic receptors in isolated strips of the ventral aorta and bulbus arteriosus of the rainbow trout. *Proc. West Pharmacol. Soc.*, 14:86.

93. Klaverkamp, J. F., and Dyer, D. C. (1974): Autonomic receptors in isolated rainbow trout vasculature. *Eur. J. Pharmacol.*, 28:25–34.

94. Klaverkamp, J. F., and Hobden, B. R. (1980): Brain acetylcholinesterase inhibition and hepatic activation of acephate and fenitrothion in rainbow trout (*Salmo gairdneri*). *Can. J. Fish Aquat. Sci.*, 37:1,450–1,453.

95. Krawkow, N. P. (1913): Uber die wirkung von giften auf die gefasse isolierter fischkiemen. *Pfluger Arch. Physiolog.*, 151:583–603.

96. Krishnamurthy, V. G., and Bern, H. A. (1971): Innervation of the corpuscles of Stannius. *Gen. Comp. Endocrinol.*, 16:162–164.

97. Laffont, J., and Labat, R. (1966): Action de l'adrenaline sur la frequence cardiaque de la carpe commune: Effet de la temperature du milieu sur l'intensite de la reaction. *J. Physiol. (Paris)*, 58:351–355.

98. Lansing, A. I. (1959): Elastic tissue. In: *The Arterial Wall*, p. 136–160. Williams and Wilkins Company, Baltimore.

99. Lochowitz, R. T., Miles, H. M., and Hafemann, D. R. (1974): Anesthetic-induced variations in the cardiac rate of the teleost *Salmo gairdneri*. *Comp. Gen. Pharmacol.*, 5:217–224.

100. Loomis, T. A. (1974): *Essentials of Toxicology*, 2nd edition. Lea and Febiger, Philadelphia.
101. Lunn, C. R., Towes, D. P., and Pree, D. J. (1976): Effects of three pesticides on respiration, coughing, and heart rates of rainbow trout (*Salmo gairdneri* Richardson). *Can. J. Zool.*, 54:214–219.
102. Lutz, B. R. (1930*a*): The effect of adrenalin on the auricle of elasmobranch fishes. *Am. J. Physiol.*, 94:135–139.
103. Lutz, B. R. (1930*b*): Reflex cardiac and respiratory inhibition in the elasmobranch *Scyllium canicula*. *Biol. Bull.*, 59:170–178.
104. Lutz, B. R. (1930*c*): The innervation of the heart of the elasmobranch *Scyllium canicula*. *Biol. Bull.*, 59:211–216.
105. Lutz, B. R. (1930*d*): The visceral afferent pathway in the elasmobranch *Scyllium canicula*. *Biol. Bull.*, 59:217–221.
106. MacDonald, A. D. (1925): Action of adrenaline on the perfused fish heart. *Q. J. Exp. Physiol.*, 15:69–80.
107. MacKay, M. E. (1931): The action of some hormones and hormone-like substances on the circulation in the skate. *Contrib. Canad. Biol. Fisheries*, New Series, 7:19–29.
108. Maetz, J. (1974): Aspects of adaptation to hypoosmotic and hyperosmotic environments. In: *Biochemical and Biophysical Perspectives in Marine Biology*, Vol. I, edited by D. C. Malins and J. R. Sargent, pp. 1–167. Academic Press, New York.
109. Majewski, H. S., and Giles, M. A. (1981): Cardiovascular-respiratory responses of rainbow trout (*Salmo gairdneri*) during chronic exposure to sublethal concentrations of cadmium. *Water Research*, 15:1,211–1,217.
110. Majewski, H. S., Klaverkamp, J. F., and Scott, D. P. (1978): Acute lethality, and sublethal effects of acetone, ethanol, and propylene glycol on the cardiovascular and respiratory systems of rainbow trout (*Salmo gairdneri*). *Water Res.*, 12:217–221.
111. McWilliam, J. A. (1885): On the structure and rhythm of the heart in fishes, with especial reference to the heart of the eel. *J. Physiol.*, 6:192–245.
112. Mott, J. C. (1950): Radiological observations on the cardiovascular system in *Anguilla anguilla*. *J. Exp. Biol.*, 27:324–332.
113. Mott, J. C. (1951): Some factors affecting the blood circulation in the common eel (*Anguilla anguilla*). *J. Physiol.*, 114:387–398.
114. Mott, J. C. (1957): The cardiovascular system. In: *The Physiology of Fishes*, Vol. I, edited by M. Brown, pp. 81–108. Academic Press, New York.
115. Murdough, H. V., Robin, E. D., Millen, J. E., and Drewry, W. F. (1965): Cardiac output determinations by the dye-dilution method in *Squalus acanthias*. *Am. J. Physiol.*, 209:723–726.
116. Nagai, M., and Iriki, M. (1978): Body colour response of the carp (*Cyprinus carpio*) during asphyxia. *Jap. J. Physiol.*, 28:265–273.
117. Nakano, T., and Tomlinson, N. (1967): Catecholamine and carbohydrate concentrations in rainbow trout (*Salmo gairdneri*) in relation to physical disturbance. *J. Fish Res. Board Canada*, 24:1,701–1,715.

118. Nakao, T. (1978): An electron microscopic study of the cavernous bodies in the lamprey gill filaments. *Am. J. Anat.*, 151:319–336.
119. Nakao, T., and Uchinomiya, K. (1978): A study on the blood vascular system of the lamprey gill filament. *Am. J. Anat.*, 151:239–264.
120. Nilsson, S. (1972): Autonomic vasomotor innervation in the gas gland of the swimbladder of a teleost (*Gadus morhua*). *Comp. Gen. Pharmacol.*, 3:371–375.
121. Nilsson, S., Abrahamsson, T., and Grove, D. J. (1976): Sympathetic nervous control of adrenaline release from the head kidney of the cod *Gadus morhua*. *Comp. Biochem. Physiol.*, 55C:123–127.
122. Nilsson, S., Holmgren, S., and Grove, D. J. (1975): Effects of drugs and nerve stimulation on the spleen and arteries of two species of dogfish, *Scyliorhinus canicula* and *Squalus acanthias*. *Acta Physiol. Scand.*, 95:219–230.
123. Opdyke, D. F., and Holcombe, R. F. (1978): Effect of angiotensins and epinephrine on vascular resistance of isolated dogfish gut. *Am. J. Physiol.*, 234:R196–R200.
124. Ostlund, E. (1954): The distribution of catecholamines in lower animals and their effect on the heart. *Acta Physiol. Scand.*, 31:1–67.
125. Ostlund, E., and Fange, R. (1962): Vasodilation by adrenaline and noradrenaline, and the effects of some other substances on perfused fish gills. *Comp. Biochem. Physiol.*, 5:307–309.
126. Perrine, D., and Georges, P. (1978): Activité de l'acetylcholine sur le ventricule du coeur de Poisson rouge *Carassius auratus*, Téléostéen, Cyprinidé. Modification de la résponse en fonction de la température. *C. R. Soc. Biol.*, 172:58–66.
127. Pettersson, K., and Nilsson, S. (1979): Nervous control of the branchial vascular resistance of the Atlantic cod *Gadus morhua*. *J. Comp. Physiol.*, 129:179–183.
128. Peyraud-Waitzenegger, M. (1979): Simultaneous modifications of ventilation and arterial PO$_2$ by catecholamines in the eel *Anguilla anguilla* L.: Participation of $\alpha$ and $\beta$ effects. *J. Comp. Physiol.*, 129:343–354.
129. Pfuderer, P., and Francis, A. A. (1975): Phthalate esters: Heart rate depressors in the goldfish. *Bull. Environ. Contam. Toxicol.*, 13:275–279.
130. Pfuderer, P., Janzen, S., and Rainey, Jr., W. T. (1975): The identification of phthalic acid esters in the tissues of cyprinodon fish and their activity as heart rate depressors. *Environ. Res.*, 9:215–223.
131. Pfuderer, P., Williams, P., and Francis, A. A. (1974): Partial purification of the crowding factor from *Carassius auratus* and *Cyprinus carpio*. *J. Exp. Zool.*, 187:375–382.
132. Pic, P., Mayer-Gostan, N., and Maetz, J. (1974): Branchial effects of epinephrine in the seawater-adapted mullet. I. Water permeability. *Am. J. Physiol.*, 226:698–702.
133. Pic, P., Mayer-Gostan, N., and Maetz, J. (1975): Branchial effects of epinephrine in the seawater-adapted mullet. II. Na and Cl extrusion. *Am. J. Physiol.*, 228:441–447.

134. Pickford, G. E., Srivastava, A. K., Slicher, A. M., and Pang, P. K. T. (1971): The stress response in the abundance of circulating leucocytes in the killifish *Fundulus heteroclitus*. II. The role of catecholamines. *J. Exp. Zool.*, 177:97–108.
135. Pohla, H., Lametschwandtner, A., and Adam, H. (1977): Die vaskularisation der kiemen von *Myxine glutionosa* L. (Cyclostomata). *Zool. Scripta*, 6:331–341.
136. Pool, C. A., and Satchell, G. H. (1979): Nociceptors in the gills of the dogfish *Squalus acanthias*. *J. Comp. Physiol.*, 130:1–7.
137. Priede, I. G. (1974): The effect of swimming activity and section of the vagus nerves on heart rate in rainbow trout. *J. Exp. Biol.*, 60:305–319.
138. Randall, D. J. (1966): The nervous control of cardiac activity in the tench (*Tinca tinca*) and the goldfish (*Carrassius auratus*). *Physiol. Zool.*, 39:185–192.
139. Randall, D. J. (1968): Functional morphology of the heart in fishes. *Am. Zool.*, 8:179–189.
140. Randall, D. J. (1970a): The circulatory system. In: *Fish Physiology*, Vol. IV, edited by W. S. Hoar and D. J. Randall, pp. 133–172. Academic Press, New York.
141. Randall, D. J. (1970b): Gas exchange in fish. In: *Fish Physiology*, Vol. IV, edited by W. S. Hoar and D. J. Randall, pp. 253–292. Academic Press, New York.
142. Randall, D. J., Baumgarten, D., and Malyusz, M. (1972): The relationship between gas and ion transfer across the gills of fishes. *Comp. Biochem. Physiol.*, 41A:629–637.
143. Randall, D. J., and Shelton, G. (1963): The effects of changes in environmental gas concentrations on the breathing and heart rate of teleost fish. *Comp. Biochem. Physiol.*, 9:229–239.
144. Randall, D. J., and Stevens, E. D. (1967): The role of adrenergic receptors in cardiovascular changes associated with exercise in salmon. *Comp. Biochem. Physiol.*, 21:415–424.
145. Rankin, J. C., and Maetz, J. (1971): A perfused teleostean gill preparation: Vascular actions of neurohypophysial hormones and catecholamines. *J. Endocrinol.*, 51:621–635.
146. Reite, O. B. (1969a): The evolution of vascular smooth muscle responses to histamine and 5-hydroxytryptamine. I. Occurrence of stimulatory actions in fish. *Acta Physiol. Scand.*, 75:221–239.
147. Reite, O. B. (1969b): The evolution of vascular smooth muscle responses to histamine and 5-hydroxytryptamine. II. Appearance of inhibitory actions of 5-hydroxytryptamine in amphibians. *Acta Physiol. Scand.*, 77:36–51.
148. Reite, O. B. (1970): The evolution of vascular smooth muscle responses to histamine and 5-hydroxytryptamine. III. Manifestation of dual actions of either amine in reptiles. *Acta Physiol. Scand.*, 78:213–231.
149. Reite, O. B. (1972): Comparative physiology of histamine. *Physiol. Rev.*, 52:778–819.

150. Reynolds, W. W., and Casterlin, M. E. (1978): Estimation of cardiac output and stroke volume from thermal equilibration and heartbeat rates in fish. *Hydrobiol.*, 57:49–52.
151. Richards, B. D., and Fromm, P. O. (1969): Patterns of blood flow through filaments and lamellae of isolated-perfused rainbow trout (*Salmo gairdneri*) gills. *Comp. Biochem. Physiol.*, 29:1,063–1,070.
152. Richards, B. D., and Fromm, P. O. (1970): Sodium uptake by isolated-perfused gills of rainbow trout (*Salmo gairdneri*). *Comp. Biochem. Physiol.*, 33:303–310.
153. Roach, M. R., and Burton, A. C. (1957): The reason for the shape of the distensibility curves of arteries. *Can. J. Biochem. Physiol.*, 35:681–690.
154. Rommel, Jr., S. A. (1973): A simple method for recording fish heart and operculum beats without the use of implanted electrodes. *J. Fish Res. Board Can.*, 30:693–694.
155. Saito, T. (1973): Effects of vagal stimulation on the pacemaker action potentials of carp heart. *Comp. Biochem. Physiol.*, 44A:191–199.
156. Saito, T., and Tenma, K. (1976): Effects of left and right vagal stimulation on excitation and conduction of the carp heart (*Cyprinus cerpio*). *J. Comp. Physiol.*, 111:39–53.
157. Santer, R. M. (1977): Monoaminergic nerves in the central and peripheral nervous systems of fishes. *Gen. Pharmacol.*, 8:157–172.
158. Satchell, G. H. (1971): *Circulation in Fishes*, (Cambridge Monographs in Experimental Biology, No. 18). Cambridge University Press, London.
159. Satchell, G. H. (1978): Microcirculation in Fishes. In: *Microcirculation*, Vol. 2, edited by G. Kaley and B. M. Altura, pp. 619–647. University Park Press, Baltimore.
160. Saunders, R. L. (1961): The irrigation of the gills in fishes. I. Studies of the mechanism of branchial irrigation. *Can. J. Zool.*, 39:637–653.
161. Sawyer, W. H. (1970): Vasopressor, diuretic, and natriuretic responses by lungfish to arginine vasotocin. *Am. J. Physiol.*, 218:1,789–1,794.
162. Schaumburg, F. D., Howard, T. E., and Walden, C. C. (1967): A method to evaluate the effects of water pollutants on fish respiration. *Water Res.*, 1:731–737.
163. Schievelbein, H., Vogel, R., and Loreny, W. (1969): Contributions to the evolution of blood pressure regulation. I. The effect of biogenic amines and nicotine on the blood pressure of fish. *Z. Klin. Chem. Klin. Biochem.*, 7:461–463.
164. Schwartz, S. L., and Borzelleca, J. F. (1968): Adrenergic responses in the shark. *Toxicol. Appl. Pharmacol.*, 12:307–308.
165. Schwartz, S. L., and Borzelleca, J. F. (1969): Adrenergic blood pressure responses in the shark. *Science*, 163:395–397.
166. Shuttleworth, T. J. (1978): The effect of adrenaline on potentials in the isolated gills of the flounder (*Platichthys flesus* L.). *J. Comp. Physiol.*, 124:129–136.
167. Skidmore, J. F. (1970): Respiration and osmoregulation in rainbow trout with gills damaged by zinc sulphate. *J. Exp. Biol.*, 52:481–494.

168. Slooff, W. (1979): Detection limits of a biological monitoring system based on fish respiration. *Bull. Environ. Contam. Toxicol.*, 23:517–523.
169. Smart, G. R. (1978): Investigations of the toxic mechanisms of ammonia to fish—Gas exchange in rainbow trout (*Salmo gairdneri*) exposed to acutely lethal concentrations. *J. Fish Biol.*, 12:93–104.
170. Smith, D. G. (1977): Sites of cholinergic vasoconstriction in trout gills. *Am. J. Physiol.*, 233:R222–R229.
171. Smith, D. G. (1978): Neural regulation of blood pressure in rainbow trout (*Salmo gairdneri*). *Can. J. Zool.*, 56:1,678–1,683.
172. Smith, D. G., and Gannon, B. J. (1978): Selective control of branchial arch perfusion in an air-breathing Amazonian fish *Hoplerythrinus unitaeniatus*. *Can. J. Zool.*, 56:959–964.
173. Sokabe, H., Oide, H., Ogawa, M., and Utida, S. (1973): Plasma renin activity in Japanese eels (*Anguilla japonica*) adapted to seawater or in dehydration. *Gen. Comp. Endocrinol.*, 21:160–167.
174. Somlyo, A. V., and Somlyo, A. P. (1968): Vasotocin-magnesium interaction in vascular smooth muscle of the hagfish (*Eptatretus stoutii*). *Comp. Biochem. Physiol.*, 24:267–270.
175. Sparks, R. E., Cairns, Jr., J., McNabb, R. A., and Suter, II, G. (1972): Monitoring zinc concentrations in water using the respiratory response of bluegills (*Lepomis macrochirus* Rafinesque). *Hydrobiol.*, 40:361–369.
176. Spoor, W. A., Neiheisel, T. W., and Drummond, R. A. (1971): An electrode chamber for recording respiratory and other movements of free-swimming animals. *Trans. Am. Fish Soc.*, 100:22–28.
177. St. Helgason, S., and Nilsson, S. (1973): Drug effects on pre- and post-branchial blood pressure and heart rate in a free-swimming marine teleost, *Gadus morhua. Acta Physiol. Scand.*, 88:533–540.
178. Steen, J. B., and Kruysse, A. (1964): The respiratory function of teleostean gills. *Comp. Biochem. Physiol.*, 12:127–142.
179. Strange, J. R., Dean, J. W., Dorman, G. K., and Fletcher, D. J. (1975): New method for recording heart and respiratory rates in catfish. *Sci. Biol.*, 1:17–18.
180. Strange, J. R., Fletcher, D. J., and Allred, P. M. (1978): Cardiac and opercular responses in channel catfish (*Ictalurus punctatus*) exposed to high levels of phosphate. *J. Environ. Sci. Health*, A13:501–515.
181. Stray-Pedersen, S. (1970): Vascular responses induced by drugs and by vagal stimulation in the swimbladder of the eel *Anguilla vulgaris. Comp. Gen. Pharmacol.*, 1:358–364.
182. Taylor, A. A., and Davis, J. O. (1971): Effects of carp kidney extracts and angiotensin II on adrenal steroid secretion. *Am. J. Physiol.*, 221:652–657.
183. Taylor, E. W., Short, S., and Butler, P. J. (1977): The role of the cardiac vagus in the response of the dogfish *Scyliorhinus canicula* to hypoxia. *J. Exp. Biol.*, 70:57–75.
184. Taylor, M. G. (1964): Wave travel in arteries and the design of the cardiovascular system. In: *Pulsatile Blood Flow*, edited by E. O. Attinger. McGraw-Hill, New York.

185. Unsicker, K., Polonius, T., Lindmar, R., Lindmar, K., Löffelholz, K., and Wolf, U. (1977): Catecholamines and 5-hydroxytryptamine in corpuscles of Stannius of the salmonid *Salmo irideus* L. A study correlating electron microscopical, histochemical and chemical findings. *Gen. Comp. Endocrinol.*, 31:121–132.

186. Vincenzi, F. F., and West, T. C. (1963): Release of autonomic mediators in cardiac tissue by direct subthreshold electrical stimulation. *J. Pharmacol. Exp. Ther.*, 141:185–194.

187. Vogel, R., Schievelbein, H., Loreny, W., and Werle, E. (1969): Contributions to the evolution of blood pressure regulation. II. Evidence for the absence of kinin-like polypeptides released by proteolytic enzymes for blood pressure regulation in fish. *Z. Klin. Chem. u. Klin. Biochem.*, 7:764–766.

188. Vogel, W. O. P. (1978): Arteriovenous anastomoses in the afferent region of trout gill filaments (*Salmo gairdneri* Richardson, Teleostei). *Zoomorphologie*, 90:205–212.

189. Wahlquist, I., and Nilsson, S. (1977): The role of sympathetic fibres and circulating catecholamines in controlling the blood pressure and heart rate in the cod *Gadus morhua. Comp. Biochem. Physiol.*, 57C:65–67.

190. Wahlquist, I., and Nilsson, S. (1979): Effects of "physiological" concentrations of adrenaline on perfused fish gills. *Acta Physiol. Scand.*, 105:37A–38A.

191. Walden, C. C., Howard, T. E., and Froud, G. C. (1970): A quantitative assay of the minimum concentrations of kraft mill effluents which affect fish respiration. *Water Res.*, 4:61–68.

192. Watson, A. D., and Cobb, J. L. S. (1979): A comparative study on the innervation and the vascularization of the bulbus arteriosus in teleost fish. *Cell Tissue Res.*, 196:337–346.

193. White, F. N. (1978): Comparative aspects of vertebrate cardiorespiratory physiology. *Ann Rev. Physiol.*, 40:471–499.

194. Wilber, C. G., and Sudak, F. N. (1960): Some effects of lysergic acid diethylamide on circulation in elasmobranchs. *Biol. Bull.*, 119:349–350.

195. Wood, C. M. (1974a): A critical examination of the physical and adrenergic factors affecting blood flow through the gills of the rainbow trout. *J. Exp. Biol.*, 60:241–265.

196. Wood, C. M. (1974b): Mayer waves in the circulation of a teleost fish. *J. Exp. Zool.*, 189:267–274.

197. Wood, C. M. (1975): A pharmacological analysis of the adrenergic and cholinergic mechanisms regulating branchial vascular resistance in the rainbow trout (*Salmo gairdneri*). *Can. J. Zool.*, 53:1,569–1,577.

198. Wood, C. M. (1976): Pharmacological properties of the adrenergic receptors regulating systemic vascular resistance in the rainbow trout. *J. Comp. Physiol.*, 107:211–228.

199. Wood, C. M. (1977): Cholinergic mechanisms and the response to ATP in the systemic vasculature of the rainbow trout. *J. Comp. Physiol.*, 122:325–345.

200. Wood, C. M., McMahon, B. R., and McDonald, D. G. (1978): Oxygen exchange and vascular resistance in the totally perfused rainbow trout. *Am. J. Physiol.*, 234:R201–R208.
201. Wood, C. M., and Shelton, G. (1975): Physical and adrenergic factors affecting systemic vascular resistance in the rainbow trout. A comparison with branchial vascular resistance. *J. Exp. Biol.*, 63:505–523.
202. Wyman, L. C., and Lutz, B. R. (1932): The effect of adrenalin on the blood pressure of the elasmobranch *Squalus acanthias*. *Biol. Bull.*, 62:17–22.
203. Yamauchi, A., and Burnstock, G. (1968): An electron microscopic study on the innervation of the trout heart. *J. Comp. Neurol.*, 132:567–587.

*Aquatic Toxicology*, edited by Lavern J. Weber,
Raven Press, New York © 1982.

# Hepatic Toxicology of Fishes

## William H. Gingerich

*National Fishery Research Laboratory, La Crosse, Wisconsin 54601*

Damage to hepatic parenchymal tissue has been the most frequently reported pathological effect in fishes exposed to various
chemical agents (30,96,129,180). The primary characteristics of this
response include vacuolation of parenchymal cells and increased
degenerative changes of hepatocytes that result in focal or zonal
necrosis. These observations support the contention that, as in mammals, the liver of fish is susceptible to damage from a variety of
toxicants. Current interest in and awareness of the role of the fish
liver in mediating processes of biotransformation and elimination
of xenobiotic compounds, as well as observations of toxicant-induced liver damage, have provided an impetus for further study of
the comparative toxicology of this organ system in these poikilothermic vertebrates.

Processes mediating hepatotoxic responses in fishes have been
studied only superficially and, consequently, are poorly understood.
While the application of many of the principles and methodologies
of mammalian toxicology is frequently useful for providing insight
and direction to studies of the comparative hepatic toxicology of
fishes, there are difficulties with rigidly following this approach.
Numerous differences exist between mammals and poikilothermic
vertebrates with respect to the morphology, physiology, and biochemistry of the organ. These differences greatly influence the hepatotoxic responses of these two groups of animals. For example,
the unique biochemical and physiological adjustments made by poikilotherms in adapting to seasonally fluctuating temperatures may

55

alter drastically the susceptibilities of warm- and cold-adapted individuals of the same species to toxicant-induced damage from certain chemicals. In contrast, the response of homeotherms to chemical insult under similar conditions would not be expected to be altered appreciably. Similarly, perceived differences between mammals and fish in the functional capacity of the liver to take up, sequester, metabolize, and eliminate chemicals can result from differences in the structural organization of the liver lobule and microcirculation within the lobule. Hence, an appreciation of the morphological differences that exist between the mammalian liver and that of lower vertebrates is an essential element in understanding the comparative toxicology of this organ.

Variability in the functional capacity of the liver is not limited to those readily apparent differences between mammals and fishes. Fishes, as a group, are extremely diverse. They comprise in excess of 20,000 individual species that occupy a wide range of environmental niches and that extend across widely divergent evolutionary pathways. For these reasons, the gross morphological similarities of the liver among fish species do not necessarily ensure the conformity of functional processes. Thus, highly divergent functional capacities can be expected in this organ among fishes.

This chapter is intended to provide an overview of current knowledge concerning hepatotoxicity and hepatotoxic processes in fishes. Where the information permits, comparisons of anatomical and physiological aspects of this organ between mammals and fishes and among fishes have been attempted. Topics pertinent to this review that have been omitted intentionally include work in the areas of chemically induced hepatic carcinomas and characterization of the hepatic mixed-function oxidase system in fishes.

## ANATOMICAL AND FUNCTIONAL CONSIDERATIONS

### Gross Anatomy

Considerable diversity is evident in the morphology and anatomy of the hepatobiliary system among the few species of fish in which this system has been studied. Such diversity complicates the tasks of both understanding the functional physiology of this organ system and evaluating the pathological processes that result from exposure to toxic agents. Anatomical differences in the liver among representative fish species are found in the number and size of lobes, the length and position of both the cystic and bile ducts, the presence or absence of a gallbladder, and structural anomalies apparent in the architecture of the sinusoid. A prominent functional difference of this organ system is the capacity of some cartilaginous and bony fishes to store large reserves of lipids in the liver. Such anatomical and functional differences influence not only toxicological processes within the liver but may distort or mask the true physiological capacity of the organ to perform certain processes.

Despite the anatomical and functional diversity evident among the livers of fishes, the gross anatomy of the organ roughly parallels that of mammals. The livers of both bony and cartilaginous fishes are either single or multilobed organs, roughly prismatic in shape, and positioned in the left ventral quadrant of the peritoneal cavity. The anterior face of the organ abuts the pericardio-peritoneal septum. Blood is supplied to the organ from two sources. In teleosts, nutrient-rich blood is supplied under low pressure from a loosely organized portal system consisting of numerous vessels that drain the entire splanchnic region. This blood is collected into a terminal sinus that lies along the dorsal margin of the liver near the hilum and enters the liver at several points along its interior surface. Oxygen-rich arterial blood is supplied to the organ by the hepatic artery, which is a branch of the coeliaco-mesenteric artery. Unlike the circulatory system of mammals in which hepatic blood is returned to the heart via the vena cava, the blood of fish is returned directly to the heart by one or more hepatic veins that pass directly through the transverse septum and empty into the sinus venosus. The negative blood pressure that has been recorded within the sinus venosus of several species of fish (160) indicates that the blood may actually be sucked or pulled through the liver (vis a fronte) rather than being forced through by positive venous pressure (vis a tergo).

The gallbladder and extrahepatic biliary tract lie within the portal region of the liver on the right side of the peritoneal cavity and are held in position by the hepato-duodenal omentum. Multiple hepatic bile ducts empty into an elongated major duct that runs along the posterior ventral margin of the liver and empties into the duodenum just posterior to the pyloric curvature of the stomach. The cystic duct branches from the major bile duct distal to the common bile duct and serves to divert bile to the gallbladder. Numerous intra- and interspecific variations in this general arrangement can be found among fish species (23). For example, certain species, including both freshwater and marine representatives of the cod family (Gadidae), lack a gallbladder and thus presumably secrete bile continuously into the duodenum. In salmonids and some other species, the hepatic ducts anastomose to form the common bile duct within the hepatic mass. The cystic duct similarly branches within the liver and runs nearly its entire length within the organ before expanding into the gallbladder near the surface.

Liver to body weight ratios of teleosts are generally less than those of higher vertebrates. In species for which determinations of organ weights have been made, fish livers were found to comprise from 1 to 3% of body weight with relative weights greater than 2% being uncommon (39,79,109,162,169,176). Great variation in liver mass exists, however, both within and among species. Intraspecific variations in liver mass are most closely associated with differences in the rates of food consumption and the time since last feeding. In controlled feeding studies using largemouth bass (*Micropterus salmoides*), the hepatic mass of fish fed natural forage species at a ratio of 4% of body weight per day for 14 days was nearly three times (1.96% of body weight) that of fish deprived of food for the same period (0.66% of body weight) (79). In a similar study using *Tilapia mossambica*, Swallow and Fleming (176) demonstrated that the relative hepatic mass of fish deprived of food for 14 days (1% of body weight) was less than half that of well-fed fish (2.4% of body weight). Variations in the hepatic mass between treatment groups in both studies were related, in part, to differences in glycogen content. Variations in relative weight and chemical composition of the liver within a given species also occur seasonally in response to gonadal maturation (1,40,50). These changes appear to result from the effects of an increased concentration of circulating estrogen and are represented in the hepatocytes by increased concentrations of DNA and RNA, increased rates of vitellogin synthesis, and an increased lipid content (51,142,144). Enhanced liver lipid content is especially pronounced among those teleost (Gadidae and Pleuronectidae) and cartilaginous fishes (Carcharhinidae and Squalidae) that concentrate much of their energy reserves in the liver as lipid. Burger (18) reported that the liver weights of dogfish shark (*Squalus acanthias*) taken just prior to parturition in the summer ranged from 6.1 to 14.6% of whole body weight. These values are well above those found in the same species during winter. Moreover, the extractable lipid in the liver of certain sharks during gestation has been found to comprise as much as 60% of the wet mass of the organ (143). Thus, nutritional and seasonal effects can greatly influence the relative mass of the liver as well as its biochemical composition. This extra "inert" mass may greatly distort the true functional mass of the organ in studies where uptake, distribution, or clearance rates are being determined.

## Blood Supply

The liver is one of the most richly vascularized organs in fishes. Using radioiodated serum albumin, Stevens (174) estimated that the blood volume of the liver of resting rainbow trout (*Salmo gairdneri*) comprised approximately 14% of the total hepatic mass. After severe exercise, this value decreased to 10%, suggesting that the liver may act to pool blood needed in times of increased cardiac output. Despite their rich vascularization, fish livers do not appear to be well perfused. In several instances in which estimates of hepatic blood flow have been reported for fish, the results suggest that the relative rate of total hepatic perfusion is less than one-fourth that of mammals. Burger (18) estimated the hepatic blood flow in spiny dogfish to be 2.35 ml/min/kg body weight, using values derived from clearance studies with the organic anion sulfobromophthalein (BSP). Total hepatic blood flow in rainbow trout similarly was estimated to be 5.2 ml/min/kg body weight based on BSP clearance data (163). A comparison of the estimated rates of hepatic perfusion in several species of fish indicates that the organ receives a proportionately smaller percentage of cardiac output in fish than in mammals (Table 1). Even when corrected for differences in the relative hepatic mass, it is apparent that the rate of hepatic perfusion in mammals is at least twice that of fish. In light of current knowledge concerning the influence of blood flow and circulation on the functional physiology of this organ in mammals, such dramatic difference in these basic physiological parameters may further accentuate other basic differences between fish and higher vertebrates in the morphology, biochemistry, and functional physiology of the liver (187). Certainly the prolonged rates of clearance estimated for both endogenous chemicals such as taurocholate (16) and exogenous chemicals such as BSP (16,17,60,120,163) are influenced, in part, by differences in hepatic blood flow. The apparent lack of well-developed supplies of hepatic arterial blood and the reduced total hepatic blood flow in some fishes indicates that the well-defined microcirculatory or ascinar units of mammals may be considerably less organized or lacking entirely in the liver of fish.

Direct control of hepatic perfusion rates in some fishes is possible by contraction and relaxation of muscular sphincters in the hepatic veins. *In vitro* studies of hepatic vein sphincters from Lamnid sharks indicate that administration of acetylcholine causes these sphincters to contract while norepinephrine promotes their relaxation (95). Similar sphincters have been reported in carp (*Cyprinus carpio*) but do not appear to exist in the goldfish (*Carassius auratus*), another member of the same family (46).

Retrograde perfusion of the liver with physiological saline through one of the hepatic veins clears blood from only discrete areas of the liver. In rainbow trout, catfish *(Ictalurus punctatus)*, and northern pike (*Esox lucius*), retrograde perfusion of the liver through the dorsal hepatic vein clears blood from approximately the dorsal two-thirds of the hepatic mass while blood remains within the ventral third of the organ (W. H. Gingerich, *unpublished observations*).

TABLE 1. Cardiac output, estimated hepatic blood flow, and relative rate of liver perfusion in selected species of fish and mammals

| Species | Cardiac output (CO) (ml/min/kg bw)[a] | Reference | Estimated hepatic blood flow (EHBF) (ml/min/kg bw) | Reference | Relative liver perfusion rate (EHBF/CO ×100) |
|---|---|---|---|---|---|
| Dogfish shark | 26.7 | Murdaugh et al. (137) | 2.35 | Burger (18) | 8.8 |
| Rainbow trout | 80.0 | Holeton and Randall (87) | 5.15 | Schmidt and Weber (163) | 6.4 |
| Rat | 320 | Dawson et al. (34) | 66.0 | Rabinovici and Wiener (151) | 20.6 |
| Rabbit | 210 | Neutz et al. (139) | 37.0 | White et al. (186) | 17.6 |
| Dog | 180 | Thilenius et al. (177) | 43.0 | Greenway and Stark (65) | 26.7 |
| Human | 70.0 | Assali (8) | 20.0 | Meyers (134) | 28.6 |

[a]bw: Body weight.

Such clearance patterns suggest that the single lobed liver of many fish may be divided into at least two distinct "circulatory lobes" of unequal volume. Such separation of circulatory pathways in the liver may be a reflection of a primitive multilobed liver. Circulation within single lobed livers of many embryonic mammalian species is known to be similarly partitioned (187).

## Structural Organization

Functional organization of the liver in higher vertebrates seems to be intimately associated with morphological and anatomical characteristics of the organ (153). While these relationships have been defined in certain mammals, few such studies have been undertaken with fishes.

As in the mammalian liver, the afferent vascular tree in the liver of fishes and its closely associated bile ducts and ductules provide the framework of support to which the mass of parenchymal cells is connected. From its entrance at the hilum, the vascular tree branches and rebranches, giving off vessels of smaller and smaller diameter. The connective tissue of the hepatobiliary capsule that surrounds the entire organ extends inward along this supporting framework and is found among the parenchymal cells as reticular fibers (3,82,113). In mammals, tridimensional budding of terminal bile ductules and the accumulation of connective tissues around them have resulted in the uniform and recurrent hexagonal pattern seen in histological preparations of the mammalian liver (153). This symmetrical array is not readily apparent in the liver of fishes because of the seemingly random branching of the hepatic vascular tree and the relatively sparse concentration of connective tissue that constitutes the intercellular meshwork of support (82,100). More commonly, the portal tracts are found to consist only of well-developed portal vessels and bile ducts (6,66,169).

Knowledge of the basic microcirculatory unit of the liver is fundamental to an understanding of the processes that mediate toxic insult to the organ. In mammals, the classic representation of a hexagonal lobule by Kiernan (101) has been regarded by anatomists and pathologists for some time to be the basic microcirculatory unit of the liver. In this representation, each lobule is defined by a hexagonal field, the corners of which are demarcated by individual portal spaces containing a hepatic arteriole, a portal venule, and a bile duct. Blood draining from the afferent vasculature at the margin of each lobule flows inward along the sinusoidal channels, irrigating the radiating chords of parenchymal cells before draining into a central vein in the middle of the lobule. While this general representation is still used by many anatomists and pathologists, it is gradually being replaced by one which appears to be more consistent with experimental observations of the microcirculatory pathways within the liver.

Rappaport (153) described the basic microcirculatory unit of the mammalian liver in terms of discrete masses of parenchymal cells or ascini that are oriented along the longitudinal axis of the terminal afferent vessels. Each ascinus is supplied with blood by a terminal afferent arteriole and portal venule. Blood flowing from these vessels mixes within the sinusoidal channels and supplies the chords of cells within the ascinus with oxygen and nutrients. Effluent blood enters into either of two terminal hepatic venules which lie at the sides of the ascinar field. Although no physical boundaries are observed between adjacent ascini, patterns of blood flow are such that each ascinar field is uniquely perfused by its own blood supply and does not appear to mix readily with blood in adjacent ascinar fields.

Zones of biochemically and functionally heterogeneous parenchymal cells, differentiated on the basis of their proximity to the afferent blood supply, have been identified within individual ascinar units of the mammalian liver (141,167). Cells containing a high level of respiratory and cytogenic enzyme activity are found in the oxygen- and nutrient-rich zone directly adjacent to the afferent vasculature. Cells near the periphery of the ascinus appear to function in the storage of fat and glycogen (153) and have been implicated in the oxidative metabolism of xenobiotics (71). Additionally, two functionally distinct subpopulations of isolated hepatocytes have been identified on the basis of their partitioning on a continuous density gradient (41,70).

An adequate representation of the relationship between parenchymal cells, vascular supply, and the biliary system has not been established in the fish liver. Both portal tracts and hepatic venules are less numerous than those in the mammalian liver (169). The arterial contribution to total hepatic circulation also appears to be considerably less than that in mammals, since the hepatic arterioles are only infrequently observed within portal spaces (3,66,100,169). The mosaic of repeating portal triads and central veins that defines the hexagonal lobules in mammals is clearly lacking in fish (7).

Anatomically, there appears to be no well-defined relationship between portal spaces and terminal hepatic venules. Most studies mention only the lack of a well-defined lobular structure within the liver (82,100,169,183). However, in the most definitive study to date, Nopanitaya et al. (140) have reported an interdigitation of portal and hepatic venules in the liver of goldfish similar to the hepatic ascinus of a mammalian liver. More definitive studies using corrosion casting techniques and dye injection would be useful in establishing general microcirculatory relationships within the fish liver.

Unlike the mammalian liver, biochemically and functionally heterogeneous zones of parenchymal cells are not prominent within the livers of fishes. Sastry et al. (158) have reported regions of high glucose-6-phosphatase (G-6-Pase) activity confined to the centrolobular region in the liver of the catfishes *Heteropneustes fossilis* and *Barbus saphose*. High activity of G-6-Pase in this area is different from that in mammals where high activity is prominent only in the periportal region. Hinton et al. (83) have reported G-6-Pase activity uniformly distributed througout the entire liver of largemouth bass. In the most complete histochemical study of fish livers to date, Welsch and Storch (185) found that the activity of 10 different enzyme systems, including NADH and NADPH diaphorases and several lysosomal enzymes, was uniformly distributed in the livers of eight different marine species. Similarly, intracellular glycogen and lipid depots are uniformly distributed within the liver mass of a number of teleosts (20,21,72,82,83,111).

Anatomically, the livers of both teleost and elasmobranch fishes differ from those of higher vertebrates in the arrangement of plates or sheets of parenchymal cells. The livers of most fish contain sheets of parenchymal cells that are two cells thick rather than one cell thick as in mammals (47,182). Thus, the effective sinusoidal surface area of hepatocytes is approximately half that found in mammals. However, considering the relatively low rate of perfusion in the fish liver, it seems unlikely that processes of nutrient exchange or extraction should be greatly impaired. Indeed, comparison of the efficiency of hepatic extraction of BSP reveals that this process is nearly as efficient in the dogfish shark (18) as it is in the mongrel dog (22).

## Ultrastructure

Generally, the hepatic ultrastructure of most species of fish appears to conform to that observed in higher vertebrates. The greatest difference observed between the groups is the presence of intrahepatic canaliculi that seem to be unique to several species of cyprinid fishes.

In general, sinusoidal channels in fish are of two types, classified as either tubulosinusoidal or sacculosinusoidal (47). The former type, which has been observed in only a few species, consists of long, narrow, cylindrical channels that course rather evenly through the liver. The sacculosinusoidal type generally has larger sinusoidal channels that appear to be flat and rectangular in shape and that course irregularly through the hepatic mass. The width of individual sinusoids of this type varies from 5 to 15 μm (47,169), while the diameters of tubulosinusoidal channels are generally narrower. As in mammals, sinusoidal channels are lined with overlapping and heavily fenestrated endothelial cells. Nopanitaya et al. (140) have shown recently, through freeze etch techniques, that the fenestrations in the endothelial cells lining the sinusoidal channels of the goldfish are between 0.05 to 0.2 μm in diameter and occur in clusters of 15 to 35. The membrane surrounding these pores contains numerous microfilaments. The large surface area provided by these pores and the lack of a limiting subendothelial basal lamina in all teleostean fishes suggest that materials are freely exchanged between the sinusoidal and the perisinusoidal space of Disse (72,82,113,140, 183,189). Limiting basement membranes have been reported only in lampreys (10,168).

The question of whether the fish liver contains cells with phagocytic activity is still being debated. Based solely on morphological characteristics, Hinton and Pol (82) reported Kupffer cells adjacent to endothelial cells lining the sinusoidal lumens in the liver of channel catfish. Bertolini (10) identified cells in the liver of brook lamprey (*Lampetra zonadreai*) that took up phosphotungstic acid and suggested that these also were Kupffer cells. Other investigators, however, have not been able to confirm the presence of such cells in the liver of other fish species (72,100,114,140); indeed, some deny that the liver of fish is capable of any phagocytic activity (49,54,155). It is premature to speculate whether or not the livers of fishes possess cells capable of phagocyte activity with so few observations on less than a dozen species of fish.

The perisinusoidal spaces of Disse appear to be well developed in a number of teleost species and have relative volumes comparable to those found in higher vertebrates (20,36,72,82,114,140). The endothelial cells lining the lumen of the sinusoid rest unevenly on microvilli that extend 1.5 to 2 μm from the sinusoidal surface of the parenchymal cells. Fat-storing cells have been identified within the perisinusoidal spaces in the livers of channel catfish (82), goldfish (140), and rainbow trout (72). The number of microvilli observed on the parenchymal cells bordering this space has been estimated to be 15 to 20 per $\mu m^2$, a value only about one-third that found in mammals (140). In brook lamprey, the plasma membrane is distinctive from that of higher fishes in that microvilli are not present on the sinusoidal surface of the hepatocyte. Instead, they are replaced by a sparse number of infoldings of the membrane surface that form extracellular canals (10).

Hepatic parenchymal cells in most fish are relatively uniform in size and vary in shape from hexagonal in trout, channel catfish, and largemouth bass to an oval or barrel shape in goldfish. Tight junctions are most frequently encountered in regions of intercellular contact (72,114,140,183), while desmosomal junctions are observed infrequently (140). Greater extracellular volume appears to exist between adjacent hepatocytes in fishes than in mammals, and in trout, the plasma membrane bordering this intercellular region contains a higher density of microtubules than it does at the sinusoidal border (72). It has been demonstrated in rainbow trout that lipoproteins are secreted in this region of intercellular contact rather than at the sinusoidal margin as in mammals (181).

The intracellular organization of hepatocytes appears to differ little from that in higher vertebrates. Nuclei of parenchymal cells are located either centrally, as in goldfish (140), or are located near the periphery of the sinusoidal surface, as in rainbow trout and channel catfish (72,82,169). The rough endoplasmic reticulum (RER) in fish hepatocytes lies adjacent to the nucleus, and mitochondria are commonly found in association with the RER (72,82,113,140). Smooth endoplasmic reticulum (SER) is generally found peripheral to areas of glycogen deposition, but it is not as prominent as in higher vertebrates. The Golgi apparatus is well developed in the species studied (72,82,113), and is found near the canalicular pole (72,82,113,183).

The greatest diversity occurring in the hepatic ultrastructure among fishes exists in the morphology of the biliary system, where at least two distinct types of canalicular units have been identified. The first type of biliary system is morphologically similar to that of higher vertebrates, in that the canaliculi occur at the surface of the hepatocyte, and actively secrete bile into ductules which occur as grooves in the cell surfaces of adjacent hepatocytes. However, unlike the unlined primary and secondary bile ductules of mammals, the terminal biliary passages in fish contain elongated ductular cells that line the ductule and are connected directly to the canaliculi by tight junctions (72). This type of biliary system has been observed in most of the teleost species in which hepatic ultrastructure has been studied. The second type of biliary system has been identified only in several cyprinid species and is of interest because of its unique combination of intracellular canaliculi and terminal ductule cells. In this arrangement, the canaliculi, found completely within the hepatocyte, empty bile directly into the lumen of an adjacent, terminal ductule cell (19,115,140,189). Plasma membranes of the terminal ductule cell, infolded and sealed by tight junctions, form the lumen of the ductule (189). Each hepatocyte has only one canaliculus; however, the lumen formed by a single endothelial cell accepts bile from more than one hepatocyte (140,189). The convex, distal portion of the canaliculus fits into the concave portion of an adjacent, terminal ductule cell and is sealed by tight junctions at the interface of the two cells (140). Ductule cells lining the terminal biliary passages are long, thin, and spindle-shaped, and, except for numerous intracellular microfilaments running longitudinally near the lumenal surface, these cells are nearly devoid of cytoplasmic elements (82,189).

## Biliary Excretion

As in mammals, the bile of fishes appears to offer a major route of elimination for a variety of chemicals. Some compounds that have been identified in significant amounts in fish bile include physiological chemicals, drugs, dyes, pesticides, and a variety of environmental contaminants (Table 2). The number and diversity of chemicals constituting this list indicate the important role of the liver in mediating processes associated with the clearance and elimination of xenobiotics. Only recently, however, have comparative studies been undertaken for the purpose of understanding these processes.

Bile formation in fish occurs at much lower rates than in mammals. The average initial bile flow rates in elasmobranchs were reported to be 1.3 μl/min/kg body weight in dogfish shark (15,18) and 2.99 ml/day/kg in the small skate (*Raja erinacea*) (15). Similarly, average bile flow rates in rainbow trout range from 0.8 μl/min/kg to 1.5 μl/min/kg (60,163). By contrast, the average initial bile flow rates in mammals have been reported to be nearly 50 times greater (104).

Estimates of the relative proportion of bile flow attributable to bile salt dependent and bile salt independent fractions have not been made in fish. Recent observations suggest that the contribution of the latter is significant. In trout with externalized biliary fistulas, bile flow rates declined by 30% during the initial 12-hr collection period, but did not decline further during the next 12-hr period (163). Gradual depletion of the available bile salt pool during the initial 12-hr collection period could be expected to account for the decreased bile flow rate during this time, indicating that at least 70% of the bile flow may be related to the bile salt independent fraction. Denton and Yousef (38) observed that the size of the total bile acid pool in rainbow trout varied, depending on the age of the animals and the time since the last feeding. The total bile acid pool in 13-month-old, well-fed fish was $14.17 \pm 0.46$ $\mu$mole, whereas in 6-month-old, well-fed fish, this value was only $0.63 \pm 0.13$ $\mu$mole. In 12-month-old fish deprived of food for 45 days, the total bile acid pool was reduced to $7.11 \pm 1.45$ $\mu$mole or nearly half that of well-fed fish. A decrease in the size of the total bile acid pool may explain, in part, the decreased plasma clearance rates of some chemicals observed in fish deprived of food (43,59). Regardless of the processes mediating bile formation and bile flow in fish, low inherent rates of bile formation can greatly influence the rate of biliary excretion of many chemicals. Indeed, differences observed in the comparative rates of biliary elimination of BSP between mammals and fish are well correlated with individual rates of bile flow among the given species (60). This may also be true for a number of other chemicals for which transport into the bile rather than metabolism limits the rate of their biliary excretion.

The propensity of a chemical to be excreted in the bile of fish is influenced by its physical and chemical properties; namely, molecular weight and polarity. Chemicals of both low molecular weight (less than 200) and low polarity are not concentrated in fish bile, but instead are eliminated through either renal or branchial routes (88). By contrast, charged or highly polar and noncharged chemicals

TABLE 2. *Chemicals excreted into the bile of fish*

| Chemical | Species | Reference |
|---|---|---|
| *Physiological chemicals* | | |
| Bilirubin | Dogfish shark | Jansen and Arias (94) |
| | Dogfish shark | Chowdhury et al. (25) |
| Bile salts | | Boyer et al. (15) |
| | | Boyer et al. (16) |
| | | Boyer et al. (17) |
| | Skate | Boyer et al. (15) |
| | | Boyer et al. (16) |
| | Channel catfish | Kellogg (98) |
| | Rainbow trout | Denton and Yousef (38) |
| | Channel catfish | Collicutt and Eales (26) |
| Thyroxine | Brook trout | Sinclair and Eales (170) |
| | Skate | Truscott et al. (179) |
| Corticosteroids | Rainbow trout | Truscott (178) |
| *Dyes* | | |
| Phenolsulfonphthalein | Dogfish shark | Guarino and Arnold (67) |
| BSP | Rainbow trout | Gingerich et al. (60) |
| | | Schmidt and Weber (163) |
| | Dogfish shark | Boyer et al. (16) |
| | | Boyer et al. (17) |

*Drugs*

| | | |
|---|---|---|
| Penicillin | Dogfish shark | Guarino et al. (68) |

*Pesticides*

| | | |
|---|---|---|
| Bayer 73 | Rainbow trout | Statham et al. (173) |
| Carbaryl | Rainbow trout | Statham et al. (173) |
| Pentachlorophenol | Goldfish | Kobayashi et al. (106) |
| DDT | Rainbow trout | Statham et al. (173) |
| 3-Trifluoromethyl-4-nitrophenol | Rainbow trout | Statham et al. (173) |
| N-Tritylmorpholine | *Sarotherodon mossambicus* | Matthiessen (127) |

*Environmental contaminants*

| | | |
|---|---|---|
| 2,5,2',5'-Tetrachlorobiphenyl | Rainbow trout | Guiney et al. (69) |
| | | Melancon and Lech (132) |
| Naphthalene | Staghorn sculpin | Lee et al. (118) |
| | Coho salmon | Collier et al. (27) |
| | Staghorn sculpin | Lee et al. (118) |
| 3,4,-Benzo[a]pyrene | Rainbow trout | Melancon and Lech (133) |
| Phthalate esters | Rainbow trout | Glickman et al. (63) |
| Pentachloroanisole | Dogfish shark | Guarino and Arnold (67) |
| 2,4-D | Dogfish shark | Guarino and Arnold (67) |
| 2,4,5-T | | |

of greater than 600 molecular weight are excreted by other routes, of which the bile is a common route. For example, BSP (MW 827) is a high molecular weight molecule that is anionic at physiological pHs. It also is excreted predominantly in the bile of both elasmo-branch (16,17,18) and teleost fishes (60,163). Moreover, restriction of the biliary excretory pathway by surgical ligation of the cystic and common bile ducts results in plasma retention of this chemical without increasing its elimination by alternate routes (60). Between these extremes lies a range of chemicals of intermediate molecular weights (300–600 MW) and polarities that appear to be eliminated in nearly equal amounts in both the urine and bile. For a number of these chemicals, biotransformation, particularly by glucuronide conjugation, is essential in influencing the route of elimination. The anionic dye phenol red (phenolsulfonphthalein, MW 354) is excreted by the dogfish shark in nearly equal amounts in both the urine and bile (67). Less than 30% of the total phenol red residue in the bile was identified as the glucuronide conjugate, while the majority of residue was identified as the parent compound. In comparison, the polar lampricides 3-trifluoromethyl-4-nitrophenol (TFM, MW 207) and 2′,5-dichloro-4′-nitrosalicylanilide (Bayer 73, MW 266) and the fungicide pentachlorophenol (PCP, MW 266), are eliminated in nearly equal proportions in the urine and bile of fishes (2,89,106). However, in contrast to phenol red, virtually all residues of these three chemicals are present in bile as the glucuronide conjugates, implying that conjugation with glucuronide is a prerequisite for their excretion into bile. The observation by Lech (116) that *in vivo* inhibition of glucuronyl transferase activity in rainbow trout by pretreatment with salicylamide reduces both the rate of plasma clearance of TFM and the absolute amount of TFM glucuronide conjugate appearing in gallbladder bile tends to confirm the important role of glucuronide conjugation for biliary excretion of chemicals of this class. Thus, from the small amount of data available, it appears that molecular weight and polarity affect biliary elimination in fish in a manner that roughly approximates that in mammals.

Some chemicals eliminated in bile may become incorporated into a pattern of entero-hepatic cycling within the animal. In this situ-ation, the compounds may be reabsorbed from the intestinal tract into the plasma where they are again transported to the liver and resecreted into the bile. This pattern of recirculation reduces the elimination or clearance of certain chemicals and is responsible for the conservation of many biological chemicals, most notably the bile salts. In the case of toxic compounds, entero-hepatic cycling may be responsible for prolonging their effects.

Studies documenting entero-hepatic circulation in fishes are limited. Eales and his coworkers demonstrated a small amount of entero-hepatic cycling of radiothyroxine in both channel catfish and brook trout (*Salvelinus fontinalis*) (26,43). In both studies, approximately 25% of the available radiolabeled thyroxine was reabsorbed from the intestinal tract and excreted into the bile over a 24-hr period in fish that had been deprived of food for at least 2 weeks. In well-fed fish, approximately 20% of the isotope was reabsorbed. While documentation is available only for thyroxine, it is likely that numerous chemicals are conserved through the entero-hepatic cycle in fish. This is especially likely in light of the relatively high β-glucuronidase activity in the intestinal tracts of many fishes (122) and the number of chemicals that appear to be excreted by fish as glucuronide conjugates.

## FACTORS INFLUENCING TOXICITY

### Diet

Of the several factors that may act to modify the toxic effects of chemicals in the livers of fishes, diet and temperature are likely to have the most profound effects. Diet has been shown to alter the toxic response of certain halogenated hydrocarbons in the mammalian liver (107,130,166). Recent studies also suggest that the diet can influence the acute toxicity of certain chemicals to fish. Mehrle et al. (131) have shown significant differences in the acute toxicity of the pesticide chlordane to rainbow trout fed different commercial rations prior to toxicity testing. They also observed that the cumulative mortality between different groups of rainbow trout and bluegills (*Lepomis macrochirus*) exposed to dieldrin or DDT could be altered significantly when the lipotropic agent methionine was incorporated into the test diets. Thus, the quality of diet influences the acute toxic response of fishes to a particular chemical or group of chemicals.

Recent studies indicate that chemical-induced liver damage in fish also may be influenced, in part, by diet. Pfeifer et al. (149) reported significant differences in the plasma activity of the enzyme alanine aminotransferase (GPT) between groups of rainbow trout treated with $CCl_4$ after each group had been maintained for several months on different commercial diets. They concluded that some constituent in the diet had rendered the livers of one group more susceptible to $CCl_4$ intoxication. Similarly, increased levels of protein in the diet have been related to an increased incidence of hepatic carcinoma among groups of rainbow trout maintained on diets containing aflatoxin $B_1$ (AFB) (117). This effect appears to be attributable, in part, to the modulatory effect of high protein diet on the activities of specific, xenobiotic, metabolizing enzymes. In trout, AFB requires metabolic activation for conversion to its ultimate carcinogenic species, which is believed to be a 2,3-epoxide derivative. Generation of this metabolite is associated with the activity of aldrin epoxidase, while its metabolic degradation is thought to involve metabolism by epoxide hydrase and glutathione-S-epoxide transferase (164). Stott and Sinnhuber (175) have shown that rainbow trout maintained on high protein diets and challenged with AFB accumulated higher liver concentrations of AFB metabolites and had lower hepatic activities of epoxide hydrase and glutathione-S-epoxide transferase than did those fish maintained on moderate or low protein diets. The enhanced incidence of primary hepatic carcinoma among trout fed diets high in protein therefore appears to be related both to the creation of an enhanced pool of AFB metabolites in the liver and to reduced capacity of the liver to readily inactivate the carcinogenic species. These observations suggest that the quality of the diet can exert a considerable influence on the susceptibility of the liver to damage by certain toxicants.

## Temperature

The unique capacity of poikilothermic organisms to adapt to eury-thermal conditions has long been recognized; however, the phys-iological and biochemical mechanisms by which this adaptation is possible have been investigated only recently (77). As discussed by Hochachka and Somero (86), biochemical mechanisms of thermal compensation may be accomplished in one or a combination of ways that involve changing either the type or quantity of macromolecules in an adaptive manner. Regardless of the mechanism by which this is accomplished, thermal compensation provides for the continuance of critical biochemical and physiological processes over a wide range of ambient temperatures.

Thermal adaptation in ectothermic organisms is accompanied by dramatic changes in the rates and routes of general metabolism. In cold-adapted animals there are marked increases in the rates of oxygen consumption and the utilization of both the pentose-phos-phate pathway and the citric acid cycle (35,85,97). These metabolic adjustments appear to allow the animal to take advantage of the increased dissolved oxygen found in cold waters. Conversely, in animals adapted to warm temperatures, utilization of the glycolytic pathway predominates (45).

Cold acclimation also results in rate increases in the synthesis of nonspecific proteins in a variety of species (33,36,75). These in-creases do not appear to be tissue specific, since increased rates of protein synthesis have been documented in subcellular fractions from muscle, gill, and liver tissues of goldfish acclimated to the cold (32).

Alteration of lipid metabolism is a basic response in thermal compensation that is predominantly associated with changes in both the quality and quantity of lipids incorporated into the membranes of the adapted animal (77). In general, the proportion of unsaturated lipids in the membranes is inversely proportional to the temperature at which the animal is adapted. Insertion of fatty acids into the primary membrane structures of cold-acclimated animals purport-edly helps to maintain the fluidity of the membrane by reducing the tendency of the fatty acids to crystallize. These membrane changes are most pronounced in organs such as the brain, gills, and liver, which have a high inherent rate of metabolic activity. Increased rates of lipogenesis and distinct increases in the proportion of unsaturated fatty acids of the linolenic acid group have been reported in the livers of cold-adapted rainbow trout (76,78). Similar observations have been made in acclimation studies of liver tissue from goldfish (4,105,119) and carp (53,188).

What influence do these metabolic adjustments to temperature exert on the response of poikilotherms to chemical toxicants? While this question has not been examined in detail, it is not unreasonable to assume that any reorganization of the rates and routes of metabolism within an organism will alter the response of that animal to specific toxicants. Biochemical adjustments of metabolism to temperature may also result in differences in the toxic response elicited by cold- and warm-adapted organisms exposed to the same toxicant. This has been demonstrated with certain specific metabolic poisons in various tissues from poikilotherms. Rates of oxygen consumption in trout muscle from warm-adapted fish were inhibited to a greater extent by treatment with iodoacetic acid than were those from cold-adapted fish, presumably because of the increased rate of utilization of the glycolytic pathway in the warm-adapted animals (85). Conversely, respiratory rates in the livers of cold-acclimated goldfish were more sensitive to the respiratory inhibitors amytal, azide, and cyanide (97). A greater percentage of unsaturated fatty acids also may be a factor, whereby cold-adapted fish could be more susceptible than warm-adapted species to toxic insult from certain chemicals. One mechanism to explain an increase in susceptibility is that $\alpha$-methylene carbons of unsaturated fatty acids are especially vulnerable to peroxidative attack by a variety of chemicals (37). Therefore, the intensity of the toxic response may be enhanced among cold-adapted organisms exposed to chemicals in which highly reactive-free radicals are suspected of mediating the toxic response, since their membranes contain a greater proportion of sites available for attack.

Thus, as in mammalian studies, control of diet and environment are essential before an understanding of toxicological processes in fish livers can be achieved.

## METHODS TO EVALUATE LIVER FUNCTION

The accurate assessment of liver toxicity in fishes has been hindered by the lack of application of appropriate clinical tools. Virtually all of the methods now being used in studies with fish have been adapted from procedures developed for use in laboratories of clinical medicine or mammalian toxicology. Basic differences in the anatomy, physiology, and biochemistry between homeotherms and poikilotherms make it imperative that such clinical methods be carefully evaluated for their potential applicability to studies with fish before they can be considered of diagnostic value in assessing fish health. In many past studies, this was not done or was done indiscriminately, leaving the validity of the results of much experimental work in question.

Tests to diagnose liver damage or dysfunction may be considered to be of two general categories: (a) those that monitor changes in physiological chemicals associated with liver function, and (b) those that test the functional capacity of the organ by monitoring the rate at which the organ clears or detoxifies exogenously administered chemicals. Of the two categories, tests of the former type have been used most frequently to screen for liver damage in fishes. Tests included in this category are those that monitor changes in the activities of tissue-specific enzymes in the plasma, those that monitor changes in biological chemicals that are metabolized in large part by the liver (e.g., bilirubin), and those tests that monitor changes in plasma proteins, such as albumin, that are synthesized exclusively or predominantly by the liver. The rationale for tests of this type is based on the supposition that the plasma concentration or activity of a particular biological chemical is increased or decreased as a result of damage to the organ.

The second type of test involves following the fate of a chemical that is specifically processed by the liver. The efficiency with which the organ metabolizes or excretes the test chemical thus provides an overall index of the functional capacity of the organ to perform a particular task. Examples of this type of test include determining plasma clearance rates for dyes specifically eliminated by the liver such as rose bengal, indocyanine green, or BSP. Other tests include determining the rate of hippuric acid formation from benzoic acid and glycine.

## Plasma Enzymes

Changes in the activity of specific plasma enzymes have been most frequently used to identify and evaluate toxicant-induced damage in fishes (24,92,93,112,124). While changes in the activity of serum enzymes have been documented in fishes following exposure to a variety of toxic substances, other factors also appear to influence these enzyme responses. Changes in serum or plasma enzymes in fish have been observed following the stress of handling and capture (11,12,13,14), from thermal stress (161), and from disease (152). Thus, while these studies indicate that certain of these plasma enzymes may provide an index of stress in fish, they contribute little to an understanding of the pathological processes associated with the stress. For plasma enzyme tests to be of diagnostic value in identifying specific organ damage or dysfunction, they should ideally fulfill criteria of tissue specificity and sensitivity.

To assure tissue or organ specificity in a test, the activity of an enzyme should be relatively high in the tissue of interest and principally confined to that tissue. Moreover, to assure that the enzyme is a sensitive indicator of pathological processes, the ratio of enzyme activity in tissue to that in the plasma should be high, so that small units of enzyme activity entering the plasma from the tissue add markedly to the total plasma activity. Sensitivity is further enhanced if the enzyme is found free in the cytoplasm and, therefore, in a form more readily diffusible into the plasma rather than bound to cellular constituents.

Of the enzymes used to assess liver toxicity in mammals, several have been evaluated using fish and appear to have application in fishery research. The aminotransferases aspartate aminotransferase (GOT) and alanine aminotransferase (GPT) appear to be useful for diagnostic applications to research in fish toxicology studies, particularly for the evaluation of lesions of hepatic parenchymal tissue. The activities of both enzymes are high in liver tissue of salmonid fishes (9,57,124,145) and, as in mammals, activity appears to be confined principally to the cytoplasmic fraction of liver homogenates (9). In addition to the liver, high activities of GOT are found in heart tissue (9,57) and erythrocytes (148). In rainbow trout, the kidney appears to be the only other major soft organ with high GPT activity (57,148). Thus, both GOT and GPT enzymes appear to satisfy criteria of tissue specificity. Unlike GPT, however, in rainbow trout the liver to plasma enzyme activity ratio of GOT is relatively low and, therefore, does not offer the sensitivity of GPT in discriminating between liver damage and damage induced in other tissues (145,152).

Other enzyme systems have failed to demonstrate adequate correlations between hepatic damage and increased plasma enzyme activity. Lactic acid dehydrogenase (LDH) activity in the plasma was increased in several species of fish following $CCl_4$ intoxication (152,156). However, LDH activity is found within many tissues in fishes, and damaged tissues other than those in the liver had likely contributed to the increase in plasma enzyme activity. Moreover, attempts to identify liver-specific LDH isozymes have not been successful (152), partly because of the numerous LDH isozymes found in fish tissues (13,125). Results of investigations with glutamate dehydrogenase (GDH), creatine phosphokinase (PK), G-6-Pase and alkaline phosphatase (AP) indicate that these enzyme systems increase little following $CCl_4$ intoxication in fish and are probably not useful in evaluating liver damage resulting from frank necrosis of the hepatic parenchymal cells (90,152). Increases in the plasma activity of isocitrate dehydrogenase (ICD) and glutathione reductase (GR) occurred in trout following treatment with $CCl_4$, but the source of these enzymes was not determined (152,172).

In mammals, changes in the patterns of certain enzymes have been used as diagnostic indices for specific types of hepatic dysfunctions resulting from acute cholestasis. These changes permit the differentiation between hepatocellular and obstructive hepatic diseases. For example, increases in the serum activities of AP, 5'-nucleotidase (5'-NT), γ-glutamyltranspeptidase (GGT), and leucine aminopeptidase (LAP), all of which are localized in the epithelial cells lining the bile ducts and in the membranes of the sinusoidal surface of hepatocytes, are found in rat plasma following extrahepatic cholestasis (110). These increases appear to result from inflammation of the lining of bile ductules and hepatocyte membranes caused by blockage of bile flow. Similar use of enzyme markers for the assessment of acute cholestasis in fish has yet to be established. A complement of enzymes similar to those found in mammals is localized in the bile ductules and sinusoidal membranes in the livers of many fishes (31,83,158,185). Gingerich (*unpublished observations*) found no change in the serum activity of either AP or GGT at 24, 48, or 72 hr after experimental ligation of the cystic and common bile ducts of rainbow trout. In a related study, the serum activities of both AP and GGT were determined from rainbow trout at 24, 48, 72, and 96 hr after treatment with the model mammalian cholestatic agent alpha-napthylisothiocyanate (ANIT) (W. H. Gingerich, *unpublished observations*). Again, no change in the serum activities of either enzyme was noted, even though the treatment resulted in significant plasma retention of BSP and appeared to greatly reduce bile flow.

## Plasma Clearance

The plasma clearance of liver-specific dyes is a well-established index of hepatobiliary function in both clinical medicine and mammalian toxicology. The rate at which these dyes are cleared from the plasma compartment is related directly to the efficiency with which the liver performs a series of functions that include extraction of the dye from the plasma, storage of dye in the hepatic parenchymal cells, biotransformation of the dye to a more polar product, and excretion of either or both the parent compound and metabolized forms into the bile. A decreased rate of plasma clearance thus serves as an indication that one or more of these processes are dysfunctioning as a result of hepatic damage and thereby have become limiting to the overall transport of dye from plasma to bile.

Recent studies have established that the processes mediating plasma dye clearance and biliary excretion of BSP in both cartilaginous and bony fishes are similar to those in mammals (16,17,60,163). These results suggest that a liver function test based on the plasma clearance of BSP may be a useful index of overall hepatic functional capacity in fishes. However, it should be recognized that, as in mammals, several factors may influence the sensitivity of this test.

Schmidt and Weber (163) demonstrated that in rainbow trout the capacity to clear BSP from the plasma is related to the dose of BSP administered. The plasma half-life of BSP in trout given doses of either 5.0 or 10.0 mg/kg (i.v.) was estimated to be 13 min, while that in fish given BSP at a dose of 15.0 mg/kg increased to more than twice that of the two lower doses (30 min). A similar dose-related increase in plasma BSP clearance has been reported in mammals and is thought to represent a temporary saturation of processes related to BSP uptake by the liver (150). Thus, the selection of an optimal dose of dye is important to ensure that hepatic function is adequately resolved by the test. The optimal dose of BSP administered for purposes of clinical evaluation of hepatobiliary processes should be one that is cleared rapidly from the plasma and yet one close to the dose necessary to exceed the clearance capacity of the liver. Doses in this range permit the resolution of minor functional changes that otherwise would be masked by the reserve capacity of the organ to clear BSP from the plasma. In well-fed rainbow trout, the optimal dose of BSP appears to be about 10.0 mg/kg, but this value is likely to vary widely among species of fish.

Food deprivation has also been shown to modify rates of BSP clearance in mammals and fishes. Plasma BSP retention and hyperbilirubinemia have been documented in mammals not fed for as few as 3 days (64). Attempts to explain these effects solely on the basis of decreased hepatic blood flow have not been successful, and impairment of processes such as hepatic dye extraction efficiency (52) or bile formation (154) have been implicated. Similarly, plasma retention of BSP has been observed in rainbow trout deprived of food for periods of 10 days or longer (59). Moreover, food deprivation has been shown to decrease the plasma clearance and biliary excretion of radiothyroxine in brook trout, rainbow trout, and channel catfish (26,42,81) and to reduce the total bile acid pool in rainbow trout (38). Thus, food deprivation may induce general, rather than specific, changes in hepatobiliary function. Such observations indicate that plasma dye clearance techniques should be used with some measure of discretion and may not be applicable to studies in which long-term exposure to sublethal concentrations of a toxicant result in reduced food consumption or anorexia among the experimental animals. Decreased hepatic blood flow (60) and high plasma concentrations of other organic anions, which may compete for biliary excretory pathways, also result in impaired plasma clearance of BSP in rainbow trout (61).

Plasma clearance of BSP has been used to evaluate liver dysfunction in fishes treated only with model mammalian hepatotoxic agents. Intoxications by both $CCl_4$ and monochlorobenzene (MCB) have been found to induce a dose-dependent plasma retention of BSP in rainbow trout (58,61). However, in both studies, the plasma activities of GOT and GPT were found to increase before plasma BSP retention was apparent, and returned to control levels only after plasma BSP clearance rates were in the range of normal values. Thus, BSP plasma clearance does not provide as sensitive an index of hepatic cell damage as do elevations of plasma enzyme activities. On the other hand, plasma clearance techniques appear to be useful in demonstrating certain other types of toxicant-induced hepatic dysfunction. Treatment with the mammalian cholestatic agent ANIT induces a significant plasma retention of BSP in rainbow trout. Gingerich (*unpublished observations*) observed plasma BSP retention as early as 12 hr after treatment with 400 mg/kg ANIT (i.p. in salmon oil) and highly significant plasma retention in all fish treated after 24 hr. Despite the evidence for impaired hepatobiliary function, serum activities of both AP and GGT remained within the range of those found for control fish, and pathological changes in both hepatic parenchymal and ductular epithelial cells were not evident by light microscopy. In this case, plasma BSP clearance appeared to offer a more useful index of hepatic dysfunction than more accepted histological and clinical diagnostic methods.

## ASPECTS OF HEPATOTOXICITY

### Histology

Evaluations of hepatotoxicity in fishes resulting from toxic agents have been made principally through histological studies. On the basis of such studies, it appears that a variety of chemicals are capable of inducing lesions in the livers of fish (Table 3). Despite the many reports of liver damage in fish following exposure to toxic agents, detailed studies of the time course for development and histological description of the hepatic lesions are found only in studies of aflatoxicosis in salmonids (73,74).

In general, the liver pathology of fishes is less diverse than that of mammals. This appears to be attributable, in part, to the relatively primitive and unstructured nature of this organ in lower vertebrates (155). The most frequently encountered types of degenerative changes are those of hydropic degeneration, cloudy swelling, vacuolation, and focal necrosis. Pyknosis, karyorhexis, and karyolysis have been reported in cases of severe intoxication. Fatty degenerative changes in fish liver are observed only infrequently in cases of chemical intoxication. In those instances when degenerative changes are observed, it is not always clear whether or not the change is a direct result of the specific toxicant. Fatty degenerative changes in fish liver have been attributable to nutritional imbalances resulting from an improper diet (135). Consistent hepatic accumulation of lipophilic vacuoles has been reported in a number of fish species following experimental intoxication with polychlorinated biphenyls (PCBs) (30,72,121,138). The accumulation of lipophilic vacuoles in hepatic parenchymal cells is also a prominent finding in experimental PCB intoxication in mammals (55).

Zonal and massive necroses are rarely observed in the livers of fishes. Pericentral necrosis has been reported in trout and catfish

TABLE 3. *Liver histopathology in fishes resulting from exposure to environmental contaminants or model mammalian hepatotoxicants*

| Class of chemical | Type of pathology | Species | References |
|---|---|---|---|
| *Heavy metals* | | | |
| Methyl mercury | Focal necrosis, capsular inflammation | Channel catfish | Kendall (99) |
| Cadmium | Enlarged lysosomes, decreased glycogen content | Carp | Koyama et al. (108) |
| Arsenic | Increased numbers of electron dense particles | Green sunfish | Sorensen (171) |
| *Industrial wastes* | | | |
| Ammonia | Pyknotic nuclei, focal necrosis, degeneration of cord array | Carp | Flis (56) |
| Phenol | Focal necrosis, vacuolization | *Clarius battrachus* | Mukherjie and Bhatta-charya (136) |
| Aroclor 1254 | Vacuolization, fatty accumulation, intracellular PAS-positive inclusions, focal necrosis | Spot | Couch (30) |
| | Irregular nuclei, increased lysosomes, vacuolization, lipid accumulation, glycogen depletion | Rainbow trout | Hacking et al. (72) Nestel and Budd (138) |

| Compound | Effect | Species | Reference |
|---|---|---|---|
| Aroclor 1254 | Increased liver lipids, inconsistent hepatomegaly, scattered foci of proliferative SER | Channel catfish | Lipsky et al. (121) |
| *Organochlorine pesticides* | | | |
| Heptachlor | Loss of glycogen and lipid content, early necrotic change | Bluegill | Andrews et al. (5) |
| Endrin | Disruption of cord array, vacuolization, focal necrosis | Cutthroat trout | Eller (48) |
| | Focal necrosis, lipid and glycogen depletion | Spot | Lowe (123) |
| | Hypertrophy of hepatocytes, pericentral necrosis | *Channa punctatus* | Sastry and Sharma (159) |
| DDT | Focal necrosis, vacuolization of cytoplasm | Brown trout | King (102) |
| | Increased SER | Guppy | King (102), Weis (184) |
| | Decreased glycogen content; decreased hepatocyte size | Zebrafish | Weis (184) |
| Dieldrin | Vacuolization, focal necrosis, disarray of cord structure | *Ophiocephalus punctatus* | Mather (126) |
| | | *Trichogaster fasciatus* | Mather (126) |
| Lindane | Vacuolization, pericentral necrosis, hypertrophy of parenchymal cells | *Ophiocephalus punctatus* | Mather (126) |
| | | *Trichogaster fasciatus* | Mather (126) |

TABLE 3. *(contd.)*

| Class of chemical | Type of pathology | Species | References |
|---|---|---|---|
| *Organochlorine herbicides* | | | |
| Dichlobenil | Focal and massive necrosis | Bluegill | Cope et al. (28) |
| 2,4-D | Glycogen depletion, PAS positive material in sinusoids | Bluegill | Cope et al. (29) |
| *Organophosphate pesticides* | | | |
| Dylox | Vacuolization of cytoplasm | Rainbow trout | Matton and LaHam (128) |
| Dursban | Fatty infiltration, vascular stasis | Sheepshead minnow | Couch (30) |
| *Model hepatotoxic agents* | | | |
| CCl₄ | Pericentral necrosis, subcapsular necrosis; hydropic degeneration, karyolysis, vacuolization | Rainbow trout | Gingerich et al. (61) |
| | Pericentral necrosis, fatty infiltration | *Heteropneustes fossilis* | Sastry and Agrawal (157) |
| | Vacuolization, focal, and laminar necrosis | Rainbow trout | Statham et al. (172) |
| Monochlorobenzene or MCB | Pericentral necrosis, hydropic degeneration | Rainbow trout | Gingerich and Dalich (58) |

which received relatively high doses of $CCl_4$ or MCB (58,61,158). The incidence of such lesions is low in fish and the time course for development (less than 6 hr) is generally much less than that for mammals. Lesions commonly observed in acute toxicity studies with $CCl_4$ include areas of diffuse focal necrosis (84,90,145) and laminar or subcapsular necrosis (61,172). The latter lesion may be the result of cellular death following direct contact of the toxicant (61) or the result of postmortem bile damage incurred during sampling (80). In either case, this lesion does not appear to be associated with the distinct centrolobular lesion characteristic of $CCl_4$ intoxication in mammals.

Ultrastructural changes have been documented in the livers of fishes exposed to certain halogenated hydrocarbon compounds or certain heavy metals. However, as in studies by light microscopy, the incidence and severity of these alterations are not as dramatic as are those in mammals exposed to the same chemicals.

Prominent ultrastructural changes have been identified in both the SER and RER in several species of fishes following exposure to a variety of organic chemicals. Reorganization of the RER from parallel to circular arrays has been observed in rainbow trout (72) and channel catfish (121) following treatment with Aroclor 1254. Focal proliferation of SER was noted in both species, as was the development of lipid inclusion bodies. Similar proliferation of RER and SER has been documented in zebra fish (*Brachydanio rerio*) and guppies (*Poecilia reticulata*) following exposure to sublethal concentrations of DDT (184) and in mullet (*Mugil cephalus*) 7 days after i.p. treatment with the inducing agent 3-methylcholanthrene (3-MC) (165). Increases in the activity of the enzyme polyaromatic hydrocarbon oxygenase were associated with these ultrastructural changes in the latter study.

Several studies have reported apparent damage to the nuclei of hepatocytes following exposure to toxic agents. Increased numbers of bizarre-shaped nuclei were observed in cells from rainbow trout exposed to sublethal concentrations of Aroclor 1254 (72) and nuclear degeneration characterized by nucleolar loss or condensation was observed following treatment with 3-MC (165). According to Hacking et al. (72), no evidence of necrosis was associated with the aberrant nuclear forms. However, Schoor and Couch (165) stated that nuclear degeneration was an early indication of cellular necrosis. A dose- and time-dependent increase in intra-nuclear electron dense particles has also been demonstrated in hepatocytes from green sunfish (*Lepomis cyanellus*) chronically exposed to sublethal concentrations of arsenic (171).

## Physiology and Biochemistry

Observations of physiological and biochemical dysfunction in fish liver have been made principally using model mammalian hepatotoxic agents. In general, these studies suggest that the physiological and biochemical changes resulting from exposure to these model toxicants are much less diverse and less severe than those found in mammals treated with similar agents. Moreover, the doses of these chemicals required to produce apparent hepatotoxic responses in fishes are nearly an order of magnitude greater than those used for comparable mammalian studies.

Liver hypertrophy is infrequently observed among fish treated with hepatotoxic agents. Gingerich et al. (61) noted that the livers of spinal-transected rainbow trout were swollen and that the fish had experienced a simultaneous gain in body weight 24 hr after receiving $CCl_4$. They attributed the hypertrophy to general edema resulting from enhanced water uptake and retention rather than from the hepatotoxic effects of $CCl_4$. A similar weight gain was noted by Pfeifer and Weber (147) in intact trout after $CCl_4$ treatment. They attributed this weight gain to renal toxicity and attendant acute oliguria produced by the $CCl_4$. Experimental intoxication of a marine fish, the yellowtail (*Seriola dorsalis*), with $CCl_4$ did not result in increased body weight. Liver to body weight ratios similarly were not altered by the treatment (156). Unlike $CCl_4$ toxicity, acute i.p. treatment with MCB does not influence water balance or liver weight to body weight ratios in rainbow trout (58). Liver hypertrophy has been reported in several estuarine and marine species following bath exposure to crude oils (44,191). These effects have been related to the induction of hepatic microsomal components by certain constituents in the oil (190).

Disruption of a number of biochemical functions in the liver of fishes is suggested by changes in plasma protein, lipoprotein, lipids, cholesterol, and glycogen concentrations following treatment with $CCl_4$. A prominent effect of experimental $CCl_4$ poisoning in fishes is a decrease in the concentration of total plasma proteins. Pfeifer and Weber (146) observed a dose-dependent decline in the plasma protein concentration of rainbow trout during the initial 24 hr following intoxication. They attributed this decrease to the dilution of proteins resulting from enhanced retention of body water and to a general loss of plasma proteins through damaged capillary beds. A significant reduction in the albumin fraction of the plasma relative to that of total plasma protein was noted 24 hr after intoxication only in those fish treated with high doses of $CCl_4$. Similar dose-related decreases in total plasma protein concentrations have been reported in rainbow trout following i.v. injection of $CCl_4$ (84) and in yellowtail (156). In both studies, a distinct decrease in the albumin fraction was confirmed through salting-out techniques and by separation and quantitation of specific protein fractions by electrophoretic techniques. Whether protein synthesis in the liver had been affected by the intoxication was not determined in any of the studies. Similar decreases in plasma protein concentration were not observed in rainbow trout following intoxication with MCB (58).

Distinct alterations in the composition of plasma lipoproteins also have been documented in fishes treated with $CCl_4$. Hiraoka et al. (84) observed a deletion of several lipoprotein bands associated with the albumin fraction in rainbow trout treated with $CCl_4$. Conversely, additional lipoprotein bands were observed in yellowtail following $CCl_4$ intoxication (156).

As in mammals, experimental $CCl_4$ poisoning in fishes results in significant changes in the lipid distribution within the body. Plasma triglyceride concentrations were decreased in several species of fish within 2 hr of dosing and remained below control values for at least 48 hr (84,156). Unlike the mammalian response to $CCl_4$ poisoning, however, liver triglyceride concentrations did not increase, and toxicant-induced fatty livers have not been reported in fish. Statham et al. (172) observed a marked decrease in the liver triglyceride concentrations of rainbow trout 2 hr after $CCl_4$ treatment. By 4 hr, triglyceride concentrations were comparable to those of control animals and remained within the limits of control animals for at least 20 hr. The failure of trout to respond to $CCl_4$ intoxication by developing a fatty liver emphasizes the physiological and biochemical differences that exist between fish and mammals in terms of the responses of this organ to toxicant insult.

Plasma activities of a number of enzymes are increased in both freshwater and marine fishes following treatment with model mammalian hepatotoxic agents (9,58,90,148,152,156,172). Comparative studies suggest that the time necessary to attain peak plasma enzyme activity in fish is less than that in mammals, but that the magnitude of peak plasma enzyme activity is reduced. Peak GOT and GPT activities in plasma of rainbow trout are detected 2 to 6 hr following intoxication with $CCl_4$, and these activities remain elevated for at least 18 hr after treatment (Table 4). Moreover, peak plasma enzyme activities of experimental fish rarely exceed those of control fish by more than a factor of 10. By contrast, peak plasma enzyme activities in mammals generally are evident from 12 to 24 hr after intoxication and the magnitude of enzyme response in laboratory mammals may be more than 50 times greater than that of the control group (103,150).

Distinct bimodal peaks in the plasma activity of GPT have been observed in rainbow trout following treatment with either $CCl_4$ or MCB. Initial increases in plasma enzyme activity were apparent within the first 4 hr after treatment with $CCl_4$ (172) and after 8 hr following MCB intoxication (58). The second peak in plasma enzyme activity was observed in both groups after 72 hr and, in the case of $CCl_4$ poisoning, appeared to correspond to a decrease in the activity of this enzyme in the liver (152).

Despite the demonstrable relationships between toxicant-induced liver damage and elevations in plasma GOT and GPT activities, little direct evidence exists to implicate the liver as the major source of the increased plasma enzyme activities in fish. *In vitro* studies

TABLE 4. *Comparison of plasma enzyme activities in several species of fish following treatment with the model mammalian hepatotoxic agent $CCl_4$*

| Species | Treatment dose (ml/kg) | Plasma enzymes | Time (hr) after treatment | | | Reference |
|---|---|---|---|---|---|---|
| | | | First increase | Maximum activity | Recovery | |
| Rainbow trout | 1.33 | GOT, GPT, LDH, GR, GDH | 6 | 6 | Elevated through 24 | Racicot et al. (152) |
| Rainbow trout | 1.0 | GPT | 6 | 12 | 24 | Pfeifer et al. (148) |
| Rainbow trout | 1.0 | GOT, GPT, ICD | 2 | 8 | Elevated through 72 | Statham et al. (172) |
| Yellowtail | 1.0 | GOT, GPT, LDH | 6 | 24 | Elevated through 48 | Sakaguchi and Hamaguchi (156) |
| Eel | 0.1 | GOT, GPT | 120 | 240 | 360 | Inui (90) |

have established that trout erythrocytes, hemolyzed by either phys-ical mixing or by exposure to $CCl_4$, contribute significantly to plasma GOT activity (145). Thus, the attendant intravascular hemolysis in rainbow trout that develops after treatment with $CCl_4$ is also likely to contribute to the elevated plasma GOT activity (61). Recent studies also implicate the kidney as a contributor, at least in part, to the increased activity of GPT in rainbow trout following $CCl_4$ intoxication. Pfeifer and Weber (147) reported that rainbow trout developed lesions in the proximal tubules and an acute oliguria accompanied by dramatic weight gains 24 hr after treatment with $CCl_4$. They suggested that renal damage induced by $CCl_4$ treatment also might contribute to plasma GPT activity. Attempts to differ-entiate between liver and kidney forms of GPT in rainbow trout on the basis of pyruvate saturation tests have not been successful (152). This leaves open the possibility that at least some of the increase in plasma GPT activity in fish treated with $CCl_4$ is contributed by damaged kidney tissue.

Perhaps the most striking evidence to indicate that the liver is the major source of GOT and GPT is that provided by Inui (90,91). In his initial studies, $CCl_4$ treatment produced histopathological lesions in the liver of eels and increased the plasma activity of GOT and GPT (90). In a second series of studies, changes in the activities of GOT and GPT in sham-operated control eels and hepatectomized eels were compared following treatment with $CCl_4$. He observed that the plasma activities of both enzymes remained essentially un-changed in hepatectomized eels, whereas those in sham-operated fish were greatly increased (91). He concluded that the liver was the primary source of these enzymes in the plasma of the eel fol-lowing $CCl_4$ intoxication.

Attempts to evaluate the nature and extent of hepatobiliary dys-function induced in fish liver by hepatotoxic agents have been lim-ited to a few studies using plasma BSP clearance as an index of toxicity. Dose-dependent plasma retention of BSP has been reported in rainbow trout following i.p. injections of either $CCl_4$ (61) or MCB (58), and in rainbow trout exposed to sublethal waterborne concentrations of MCB for 15 and 30 days (59). Results from subsequent studies suggest that plasma BSP retention induced by i.p. treatment with $CCl_4$ is due, in part, to the reduced rate of hepatic accumulation of BSP (62). Reduced hepatic blood flow or impaired hepatic extraction efficiency may both have contributed to the inability of livers from treated fish to accumulate BSP. Unlike rats poisoned with $CCl_4$, the rate of bile formation and the biliary transport maximum for BSP in trout were not affected by the treatment.

## ACKNOWLEDGMENTS

The author wishes to express his gratitude to Ms. Rosalie A. Schnick and Ms. Carol J. Bjerke for their constant help in acquiring technical materials for this manuscript and to Ms. Alice J. Haas for her enduring patience in typing its many drafts.

## REFERENCES

1. Aida, K., Hirose, K., and Yokote, M. (1973): Physiological studies on gonadal maturation of fishes. II. Histological changes in the liver cells of Ayu following gonadal maturation and estrogen administration. *Bull. Jap. Soc. Sci. Fish.*, 39:1,107–1,115.
2. Allen, J. L., Dawson, V. K., and Hunn, J. B. (1979): Excretion of the lampricide Bayer 73 by rainbow trout. In: *Aquatic Toxicology*, edited by L. L. Marking and R. A. Kimerle, pp. 52–61. American Society for Testing and Materials, Spec. Tech. Publ. 667, Philadelphia.
3. Anderson, B. G., and Mitchum, D. L. (1974): *Atlas of Trout Histology*. Bulletin No. 13, Wyoming Game and Fish Department, Cheyenne, Wyoming.
4. Anderson, T. R. (1970): Temperature adaptation and the phospholipids of membranes in goldfish (*Carassius auratus*). *Comp. Biochem. Physiol.*, 33:663–687.
5. Andrews, A. K., Van Valin, C. C., and Stebbings, B. E. (1967): Some effects of heptachlor on bluegills (*Lepomis macrochirus*). *Trans. Am. Fish. Soc.*, 95:297–308.
6. Ashley, L. M. (1967): Histopathology of rainbow trout aflatoxicosis. In: *Trout Hepatoma Research Conference Papers*, edited by J. E. Halver and I. A. Mitchell, pp. 103–120. Fish and Wildlife Service Research Report 70.
7. Ashley, L. M. (1973): Animal model: Liver cell carcinoma in rainbow trout. *Am. J. Pathol.*, 72:345–348.
8. Assali, N. S. (1967): Some aspects of fetal life *in utero* and changes at birth. *Am. J. Obstet. Gynecol.*, 97:324–331.

9. Bell, G. R. (1968): Distribution of transaminases (aminotransferases) in the tissues of Pacific salmon with emphasis on the properties and diagnostic use of glutamic-oxalacetic transaminase. *J. Fish. Res. Board Can.*, 25:1,247–1,268.

10. Bertolini, B. (1965): The structure of the liver cells during the life cycle of a brook lamprey (*Lampetra zonadreai*). *Z. Zellforsch.*, 67:297–318.

11. Bouck, G. R. (1980): Concentration of leucine aminonaphthylamidase (LAN) and soluble protein in tissues of rainbow trout (*Salmo gairdneri*). *Can. J. Fish. Aquat. Sci.*, 37:116–120.

12. Bouck, G. R., and Ball, R. C. (1966): Influence of capture methods on blood characteristics and mortality in the rainbow trout. *Trans. Am. Fish. Soc.*, 95:170–176.

13. Bouck, G. R., and Ball, R. C. (1968): Comparative electrophoretic patterns of lactate dehydrogenase in three species of trout. *J. Fish. Res. Board Can.*, 25:1,323–1,331.

14. Bouck, G. R., Schneider, P. W., Jacobsen, J., and Ball, R. C. (1975): Characterization and subcellular localization of leucine aminonaphthylamidase (LAN) in rainbow trout (*Salmo gairdneri*). *J. Fish. Res. Board Can.*, 32:1,289–1,295.

15. Boyer, J. L., Schwarz, J., and Smith, N. (1976a): Biliary secretion in elasmobranchs. I. Bile collection and composition. *Am. J. Physiol.*, 230:970–973.

16. Boyer, J. L., Schwarz, J., and Smith, N. (1976b): Biliary secretion in elasmobranchs. II. Hepatic uptake and biliary excretion of organic anions. *Am. J. Physiol.*, 230:974–981.

17. Boyer, J. L., Schwarz, J., and Smith, N. (1976c): Selective hepatic uptake and biliary excretion of $^{35}$S-sulfobromophthalein in marine elasmobranchs. *Gastroenterology*, 70:254–256.

18. Burger, J. W. (1967): Some aspects of liver function in the spiny dogfish, *Squalus acanthius*. In: *Sharks, Skates, and Rays*, edited by P. W. Gilbert, R. F. Mathewson, and D. P. Rall, pp. 293–298. The Johns Hopkins Press, Baltimore.

19. Byczkowska-Smyk, W. (1968a): Bile canaliculi in hepatic cells of the crucian carp (*Cyprinus carassius* L.) and tench (*Tinca tinca* L.). *Acta Biol. Craco. Ser. Zool.*, 11:93–99.

20. Byczkowska-Smyk, W. (1968b): Observations of the ultrastructure of the hepatic cells of the burbot (*Lota lota*). *Zool. Pol.*, 18:287–298.

21. Byczkowska-Smyk, W. (1970): The ultrastructure of hepatic cells of the carp (*Cyprinus carpio* L.) and gudgeon (*Gobio gobio* L.). *Acta Biol. Craco. Ser. Zool.*, 13:105–109.

22. Casselman, W. G. B., and Rappaport, A. M. (1954): Guided catheterization of hepatic veins and estimation of hepatic blood flow by the bromosulphalein method in normal dogs. *J. Physiol.*, 124:173–182.

23. Chakrabarte, J., Saharya, R., and Belsare, D. K. (1973): Structure of the gallbladder in some freshwater teleosts. *Z. Mikrosk. Anat. Forsch.*, 87:23–32.

24. Christiansen, G., Hunt, G., and Fiandt, J. (1977): The effects of methyl-mercuric chloride, cadmium chloride, and lead nitrate on six biochemical factors of the brook trout (*Salvelinus fontinalis*). *Toxicol. Appl. Pharmacol.*, 42:523–530.
25. Chowdhury, J. R., Chowdhury, N. R., and Arias, I. M. (1980): Bilirubin conjugation in the spiny dogfish, *Squalus acanthias*, the small skate, *Raja erinacea*, and the winter flounder, *Pseudopleuronectes americanus*. *Comp. Biochem. Physiol.*, 66B:523–528.
26. Collicutt, J. M., and Eales, J. G. (1974): Excretion and enterohepatic cycling of $^{125}$I-L-thyroxine in channel catfish, *Ictalurus punctatus* Rafinesque. *Gen. Comp. Endocrinol.*, 23:390–402.
27. Collier, T. K., Thomas, L. C., and Malins, D. C. (1978): Influence of environmental temperature on disposition of dietary naphthalene in coho salmon (*Oncorhynchus kisutch*): Isolation and identification of individual metabolites. *Comp. Biochem. Physiol.*, 61C:23–28.
28. Cope, O. B., McCraren, J. P., and Eller, L. L. (1969): Effects of dichlobenil on two fish pond environments. *Weed Sci.*, 17:158.
29. Cope, O. B., Wood, E. M., and Wallen, G. H. (1970): Some chronic effects of 2,4-D on the bluegill (*Lepomis macrochirus*). *Trans. Am. Fish. Soc.*, 99:1–12.
30. Couch, J. A. (1975): Histopathological effects of pesticides and related chemicals on the livers of fishes. In: *The Pathology of Fishes* edited by W. E. Ribelin and G. Migaki, pp. 559–584. University of Wisconsin Press, Madison.
31. Cvancara, V. A., and Huang, W. (1978): Tissue alkaline phosphatase activity in selected freshwater teleosts. *Comp. Biochem. Physiol.*, 60B:221–224.
32. Das, A. B. (1967): Biochemical changes in tissues of goldfish acclimated to high and low temperatures. II. Synthesis of protein and RNA of subcellular fractions and tissue composition. *Comp. Biochem. Physiol.*, 21:469–485.
33. Das, A. B., and Prosser, C. L. (1967): Biochemical changes in tissues of goldfish acclimated to high and low temperatures. I. Protein synthesis *Comp. Biochem. Physiol.*, 21:449–469.
34. Dawson, C. A., Nadel, E. R., and Horvath, S. M. (1966): Cardiac output in the cold stressed swimming rat. *Am. J. Physiol.*, 213: 320–335.
35. Dean, J. M. (1969): The metabolism of tissues of thermally acclimated rainbow trout (*Salmo gairdneri*). *Comp. Biochem. Physiol.*, 29:187–196.
36. Dean, J. M., and Berlin, J. D. (1969): Alterations in hepatocyte function of thermally acclimated rainbow trout (*Salmo gairdneri*). *Comp. Biochem. Physiol.*, 29:307–312.
37. Demopoulos, H. B. (1973): The basis of free radical pathology. *Fed. Proceed.*, 32:1,859–1,861.
38. Denton, J. E., and Yousef, M. K. (1974): Bile acid composition of rainbow trout, *Salmo gairdneri*. *Lipids*, 9:945–951.
39. Denton, J. E., and Yousef, M. K. (1976): Body composition and organ weights of rainbow trout, *Salmo gairdneri*. *J. Fish Biol.*, 8:489–499.

40. de Vlaming, V. L., Shing, J., Paquette, G., and Vuchs, R. (1977): *In vivo* and *in vitro* effect of oestradiol-17-β on lipid metabolism in *Notemigonus crysoleusus*. *J. Fish Biol.*, 10:273–285.

41. Drachmans, P., Wanson, J. C., and Musselmans, R. (1975): Isolation and subfractionation on ficoll gradients of adult rat hepatocytes. *J. Cell. Biol.*, 66:1–22.

42. Eales, J. G. (1979): Comparison of L-thyroxine and 3,5,3′-triodo-L-thyronine kinetics in fed and starved rainbow trout (*Salmo gairdneri*). *Comp. Biochem. Physiol.*, 62A:295–300.

43. Eales, J. G., and Sinclair, D. A. R. (1974): Enterohepatic cycling of thyroxine in starved and fed brook trout (*Salvelinus fontinalis* Mitchill). *Comp. Biochem. Physiol.*, 49A:661–672.

44. Eisler, R., and Kissil, G. M. (1975): Toxicities of crude oils and oil-dispersant mixtures to juvenile rabbitfish, *Siganus rivulatus*. *Trans. Am. Fish. Soc.*, 1,975:571–578.

45. Ekberg, D. R. (1962): Anaerobic and aerobic metabolism in gills of crucian carp adapted to high and low temperatures. *Comp. Biochem. Physiol.*, 5:123–128.

46. Elias, H. (1952): The hepatic venous throttle musculature, a mechanism harmful to the individual, but perhaps beneficial to the species. *Am. Nat.*, 87:119–120.

47. Elias, H., and Bengelsdorf, H. (1953): The structure of the liver of vertebrates. *Acta Anat.*, 19:297–337.

48. Eller, L. L. (1971): Histopathologic lesions in cutthroat trout (*S. clarki*) exposed chronically to the insecticide endrin. *Am. J. Pathol.*, 64:321–336.

49. Ellis, A. E., Munro, A. L. S., and Roberts, R. J. (1976): Defense mechanisms in fish. I. A study of the phagocytic system and the fate of intraperitoneally injected particulate material in the plaice (*Pleuronectes platessa*). *J. Fish Biol.*, 8:67–78.

50. Emmersen, B. K., and Petersen, I. M. (1976a): Natural occurrence and experimental induction by estradiol-17-β, of a lipophosphoprotein (vitellogin) in flounder (*Platichthyes flesus*, L.). *Comp. Biochem. Physiol.*, 54B:443–446.

51. Emmersen, B. K., and Petersen, I. M. (1976b): Protein, RNA, and DNA metobolism in relation to ovarian vitellogenic growth in the flounder *Platichthyes flesus* (L). *Comp. Biochem. Physiol.*, 55B:315–321.

52. Engleking, L. R., and Gornwall, R. (1979): Effects of fasting on hepatic bile acid clearance. *Proc. Soc. Exp. Biol. Med.*, 161:123–127.

53. Farkas, T., and Csengeri, I. (1976): Biosynthesis of fatty acids by the carp, *Cyprinus carpio*, in relation to environmental temperature. *Lipids*, 11:401–407.

54. Ferguson, H. W. (1975): Phagocytosis by the endocardial lining of cells of the atrium of plaice (*Pleuronectes platessa*). *J. Comp. Pathol.*, 85:561–569.

55. Fishbein, L. (1974): Toxicity of chlorinated biphenyls. *Annu. Rev. Pharmacol.*, 14:139–156.

56. Flis, J. (1968): Anatomicohistopathological changes induced in carp (*Cyprinus carpio*) by ammonia water. II. Effect of subtoxic concentrations. *Acta Hydrobiol.*, 10:225–238.
57. Gaudet, M., Racicot, J. G., and Leray, C. (1975): Enzyme activities of plasma and selected tissues in rainbow trout, *Salmo gairdneri*. *J. Fish Biol.*, 7:505–512.
58. Gingerich, W. H., and Dalich, G. M. (1978): An evaluation of liver toxicity in rainbow trout following treatment with monochlorobenzene. *Proc. West. Pharmacol. Soc.*, 21:475–480.
59. Gingerich, W. H., and Weber, L. J. (1979): Assessment of clinical procedures to evaluate liver intoxication in fish. *Ecol. Res. Ser.*, EPA (Environ. Prot. Agency)-600/3-79-088.
60. Gingerich, W. H., Weber, L. J., and Larson, R. E. (1977): Hepatic accumulation, metabolism, and biliary excretion of sulfobromophthalein by rainbow trout (*Salmo gairdneri*). *Comp. Biochem. Physiol.*, 58C:113–120.
61. Gingerich, W. H., Weber, L. J., Larson, R. E. (1978*a*): Carbon tetrachloride-induced retention of sulfobromophthalein in the plasma of rainbow trout. *Toxicol. Appl. Pharmacol.*, 43:147–158.
62. Gingerich, W. H., Weber, L. J., and Larson, R. E. (1978*b*): The effect of carbon tetrachloride on hepatic accumulation, metabolism, and biliary excretion of sulfobromophthalein in rainbow trout. *Toxicol. Appl. Pharmacol.*, 43:159–167.
63. Glickman, A. H., Statham, C. N., Wu, A., and Lech, J. J. (1977): Studies on the uptake, metabolism, and disposition of pentachlorophenol and pentachloroanisole in rainbow trout. *Toxicol. Appl. Pharmacol.*, 41:649–658.
64. Gornwall, R. (1975): Effects of fasting on hepatic function in ponies. *Am. J. Vet. Res.*, 36:147–150.
65. Greenway, C. V., and Stark, R. D. (1971): Hepatic vascular bed. *Physiol. Rev.*, 51:23–52.
66. Grizzle, J. M., and Rogers, W. A. (1976): *Anatomy and Histology of the Channel Catfish.* Auburn University Agric. Exp. Sta., Auburn Printing, Inc., Auburn, Alabama.
67. Guarino, A. M., and Arnold, S. T. (1979): Xenobiotic transport mechanisms and pharmacokinetics in the dogfish shark. In: *Pesticide and Xenobiotic Metabolism in Aquatic Organisms*, edited by M. A. Q. Khan, J. J. Lech, and J. J. Menn, pp. 233–258. ACS Symposium Series No. 99, Washington, D. C.
68. Guarino, A. M., Briley, P. M., Anderson, J. B., Kinter, M. F., Schneiderman, S., Klipp, L. D., and Adamson, R. H. (1972): Renal and hepatic excretion of foreign compounds by *Squalus acanthius*. *Bull. M. Desert Isl. Biol. Lab.*, 12:41–44.
69. Guiney, P. D., Peterson, R. E., Melancon, Jr., M. J., and Lech, J. J. (1977): The distribution and elimination of 2,5,2′,5′-[$^{14}$C]tetrachlorobiphenyl in rainbow trout. *Toxicol. Appl. Pharmacol.*, 39:329–335.

70. Gumucio, J. J., DeMason, L. J., Miller, D. L., and Keener, M. (1976): Preparation of periportal and centrilobular hepatocytes from rat liver. *Gastroenterology*, 71:910.
71. Gumucio, J. J., DeMason, L. J., Miller, D. L., Krezoski, S. O., and Keener, M. (1978): Induction of cytochrome P-450 in a selective subpopulation of hepatocytes. *Am. J. Physiol.*, 234:C102–C109.
72. Hacking, M. A., Budd, J., and Hodson, K. (1978): The ultrastructure of the liver of the rainbow trout: Normal structure and modifications after chronic administration of a polychlorinated biphenyl Aroclor 1254. *Can. J. Zool.*, 56:477–491.
73. Halver, J. E., Ashley, L. M., and Smith, R. R. (1969): Aflatoxicosis in coho salmon. *Nat. Can. Inst. Monogr.*, 31:141–155.
74. Halver, J. E., and Mitchell, I. A., editors. (1967): *Trout Hepatoma Research Conference Papers*. Fish and Wildlife Service Research Report 70.
75. Haschmeyer, A. E. V. (1968): Compensation of liver protein synthesis in temperature acclimated toadfish, *Opsanus tau. Biol. Bull.*, 135:130–140.
76. Hazel, J. R. (1979): Influence of thermal acclimation on membrane lipid composition of rainbow trout liver. *Am. J. Physiol.*, 236:R91–R101.
77. Hazel, J. R., and Prosser, C. L. (1974): Molecular mechanisms of temperature compensation in poikilotherms. *Physiol. Rev.*, 31:620–677.
78. Hazel, J. R., and Sellner, P. A. (1979): Fatty acid and sterol synthesis by hepatocytes of thermally acclimated rainbow trout (*Salmo gairdneri*). *J. Exp. Zool.*, 209:105–114.
79. Heidiger, R. C., and Crawford, S. D. (1977): Effect of temperature and feeding rate on the liver-somatic index of the largemouth bass *Micropterus salmoides. J. Fish. Res. Board Can.*, 34:633–638.
80. Hendricks, J. D., Hunter, L. H., and Wales, J. H. (1976): Postmortem bile damage to rainbow trout (*Salmo gairdneri*) livers. *J. Fish. Res. Board Can.*, 33:2,613–2,616.
81. Higgs, D. A., and Eales, J. G. (1977): Influence of food deprivation on radioiodothyroxine and radioiodide kinetics in yearling brook trout, *Salvalinus fontinalis* (Mitchill), with a consideration of the extent of L-thyroxine conversion to 3,5,3'-triodo-L-thyronine. *Gen. Comp. Endocrinol.*, 32:29–40.
82. Hinton, D. E., and Pool, C. R. (1976): Ultrastructure of the liver in channel catfish *Ictalurus punctatus* (Rafinesque). *J. Fish Biol.*, 8:209–220.
83. Hinton, D. E., Snipes, R. L., and Kendall, M. W. (1972): Morphology and enzyme histochemistry in the liver of largemouth bass (*Micropterus salmoides*). *J. Fish. Res. Board Can.*, 29: 531–534.
84. Hiraoka, T., Nakagawa, H., and Murachi, S. (1979): Blood properties of rainbow trout in acute hepatotoxicity by carbon tetrachloride. *Bull. Jap. Soc. Sci. Fish.*, 45:527–532.
85. Hochachka, P. W., and Hayes, F. R.(1962): The effects of temperature acclimation on pathways of glucose metabolism in the trout. *Can. J. Zool.*, 40:261–270.

86. Hochachka, P., and Somero, G. N. (1973): *Strategies of Biochemical Adaptation.* W. B. Saunders, Philadelphia.

87. Holeton, G. F., and Randall, D. J. (1967): The effect of hypoxia upon the partial pressure of gases in the blood and water afferent and efferent to the gills of rainbow trout. *J. Exp. Biol.*, 46:317–327.

88. Hunn, J. B., and Allen, J. L. (1974): Movement of drugs across the gills of fish. *Annu. Rev. Pharmacol.*, 14:47–55.

89. Hunn, J. B., and Allen, J. L. (1975): Residue dynamics of quinaldine and TFM in rainbow trout. *Gen. Pharmacol.*, 6:15–18.

90. Inui, Y. (1968): Pathological study on the effects of carbon tetrachloride poisoning on the eel liver. *Bull. Freshw. Fish. Res. Lab.*, 18:157–164.

91. Inui, Y. (1969): Mechanism of the increase of plasma glutamic oxalacetic transaminase and plasma glutamic pyruvic transaminase activities in acute hepatitis of the eel. *Bull. Freshw. Fish. Res. Lab.*, 19:25–30.

92. Jackim, E. (1973): Influence of lead and other metals on fish $\delta$-aminolevulinate dehydrase activity. *J. Fish. Res. Board Can.*, 30:560–562.

93. Jackim, E., Hamlin, J. M., and Sonis, S. (1970): Effects of metal poisoning on five liver enzymes in the killifish (*Fundulus heteroclitus*). *J. Fish. Res. Board Can.*, 27:383–390.

94. Jansen, P. L. M. and Arias, I. M. (1977): Bilirubin metabolism in the spiny dogfish, *Squalus acanthias*, and the small skate, *Raja erinacea. Comp. Biochem. Physiol.*, 56B:255–258.

95. Johansen, K., and Hanson, D. (1967): Hepatic vein sphinctors in elasmobranchs and their significance in controlling hepatic blood flow. *J. Exp. Biol.*, 46:195–203.

96. Johnson, D. W. (1968): Pesticides and fishes—A review of selected literature. *Trans. Am. Fish. Soc.*, 97:398–424.

97. Kanungo, M. S., and Prosser, C. L. (1959): Physiological and biochemical adaptation of goldfish to cold and warm temperatures. II. Oxygen consumption and oxidative phosphorylation of liver mitochondria. *J. Cell. Comp. Physiol.*, 54:265–274.

98. Kellogg, T. F. (1975): The biliary bile acids of the channel catfish, *Ictalurus punctatus. Comp. Biochem. Physiol.*, 50B:109–111.

99. Kendall, M. W. (1977): Acute effects of methyl mercury toxicity in channel catfish (*Ictalurus punctatus*) liver. *Bull. Environ. Contam. Toxicol.*, 18:143–151.

100. Kendall, M. W., and Hawkins, W. E. (1975): Hepatic morphology and acid phosphatase localization in the channel catfish (*Ictalurus punctatus*). *J. Fish. Res. Board Can.*, 32:1,459–1,464.

101. Kiernan, F. (1833): The anatomy and physiology of the liver. *Philos. Trans. R. Soc. London,* ser. B, 123:711.

102. King, S. F. (1962): Some effects of DDT on the guppy and the brown trout. *U.S. Fish Wildl. Serv., Spec. Sci. Rep.-Fish. 399.*

103. Klaassen, C. D., and Plaa, G. L. (1966): Relative effects of various chlorinated hydrocarbons on liver and kidney function in mice. *Toxicol. Appl. Pharmacol.*, 9:139–151.

104. Klaassen, C. D., and Plaa, G. L. (1967): Determination of sulfobromo-phthalein storage and excretory rate in small animals. *J. Appl. Physiol.*, 22:1,151–1,155.
105. Knipprath, W. G., and Mead, J. F. (1967): The effect of environmental temperature on the fatty acid composition and on the *in vivo* incorporation of 1-[14]C-acetate in goldfish (*Carassius auratus* L.). *Lipids*, 1:121–128.
106. Kobayashi, K., Kimura, S., and Shimizu, E. (1977): Studies on the metabolism of chlorophenols in fish. IX. Isolation and identification of pentachlorophenyl-β-glucuronide accumulated in bile of goldfish. *Bull. Jap. Soc. Sci. Fish.*, 43:601–607.
107. Korsrud, G. O., Kuiper-Goodman, T., Hasselager, E., Grice, H. C., and McLaughlan, J. M. (1976): Effects of dietary protein level on carbon tetrachloride induced liver damage in rats. *Toxicol. Appl. Pharmacol.*, 37:1–12.
108. Koyama, J., Fujita, M., and Itayawa, Y. (1979): Effects of oral administration of cadmium on fish. IV. Effects on ultrastructure of hepatic and renal cells of carp and porgy. *Bull. Jap. Soc. Sci. Fish.*, 45:429–436.
109. Krumholz, L. A. (1958): Relative weights of some viscera in the Atlantic marlins. *Bull. Am. Mus. Nat. Hist.*, 114:402–404.
110. Kryszewski, A. J., Neale, G., Whitfield, J. B., and Moss, D. W. (1973): Enzyme changes in experimental biliary obstruction. *Clin. Chim. Acta*, 47:175–182.
111. Kulkarni, R. B., and Belsare, D. K. (1975): Histomorphological observations on the liver in some freshwater teleosts. *Z. Mikrosk.-Anat. Forsch.*, 5:922–933.
112. Lane, C. E., and Scura, E. D. (1970): Effects of dieldrin on glutamic-oxaloacetic transaminase in *Poecilia latipinna*. *J. Fish. Res. Board Can.*, 27:1,869–1,871.
113. Langer, M. (1979a): Histological investigation of the teleost liver. I. The structure of the parenchymal cells. *Z. Mikrosk.-Anat. Forsch.*, 93:829–848.
114. Langer, M. (1979b): Histological investigations of the teleost liver. II. The blood vasculature. *Z. Mikrosk.-Anat. Forsch.*, 93:849–857.
115. Langer, M. (1979c): Histological investigations of the teleost liver. III. The biliary system. *Z. Mikrosk.-Anat. Forsch.*, 93;1,105–1,136.
116. Lech, J. J. (1973): Isolation and identification of 3-trifluoromethyl-4-nitrophenol glucuronide from bile of rainbow trout exposed to 3-trifluoromethyl-4-nitrophenol. *Toxicol. Appl. Pharmacol.*, 24:114–121.
117. Lee, D. J., Sinnhuber, R. O., Wales, J. H., and Putnam, G. B. (1978): Effect of dietary protein on the response of rainbow trout (*Salmo gairdneri*) to aflatoxin $B_1$. *J. Natl. Cancer Inst.*, 60:317–320.
118. Lee, R. F., Saurehaber, R., and Dobbs, G. H. (1972): Uptake, metabolism, and discharge of polycyclic aromatic hydrocarbons by marine fish. *Mar. Biol.*, 17:201–208.
119. Leslie, J. M., and Buckley, J. T. (1976): Phospholipid composition of goldfish (*Carassius auratus* L.) liver and brain and temperature dependence of phosphatidyl choline synthesis. *Comp. Biochem. Physiol.*, 53:335–337.

120. Levine, R. I., Reyes, H., Levi, A. J., Gatmaitan, Z., and Arias, J. M. (1971): Phylogenetic study of organic anion transfer from plasma into the liver. *Nature (London), New Biol.*, 231:277–279.
121. Lipsky, M. M., Klaunig, J. E., and Hinton, D. E. (1978): Comparison of acute response to polychlorinated biphenyl in liver of rat and channel catfish: A biochemical and morphological study. *J. Toxicol. Environ. Health*, 4:107–121.
122. Love, R. M. (1970): *The Chemical Biology of Fishes.* Academic Press, New York.
123. Lowe, J. I. (1965): Some effects of endrin on estuarine fishes. *Proc. Annu. Conf. Southeast. Assoc. Game Fish Comm.*, 19:271–276.
124. Lue-Hing, C. (1966): *Significant relationships between serum enzymes in fish and pesticide pollution detection.* Ph.D. Thesis, Washington University, St. Louis, Missouri.
125. Massaro, E. J. (1973): The lactate dehydrogenase isozymes of *Coregonus hoyi* Gill (Pices: Salmoidae): Tissue distribution, immunochemistry, and molecular weight. *Comp. Biochem. Physiol.*, 46A:353–357.
126. Mather, D. S. (1972): Histopathological changes in the liver of fishes resulting from exposure to dieldrin and lindane. *Toxicon*, 13:109–110.
127. Matthiessen, P. (1977): Uptake, metabolism, and excretion of the molluscicide N-trityl-morpholine by the tropical food fish *Sarotherodon mossambicus* (Peters). *J. Fish Biol.*, 11:497–509.
128. Matton, P., and LaHam, Q. N. (1969): Effects of the organophosphate Dylox on rainbow trout larvae. *J. Fish. Res. Board Can.*, 26:2,193.
129. McKim, J. M., Christiansen, G. M., Tucker, J. H., Beloit, D. A., and Lewis, M. J. (1974): Effects of pollution on freshwater fish. *J. Water Pollut. Control Fed.*, 46:1,540–1,591.
130. McLean, A. E. M., and McLean, E. K. (1966): The effect of diet and 1,1,1-tricholoro-2,2-bis-(p-chlorophenyl)ethane (DDT) on microsomal hydroxylating enzymes and on sensitivity of rats to carbon tetrachloride poisoning. *Biochem. J.*, 100:564–571.
131. Mehrle, P. M., Mayer, F. L., and Johnson, W. W. (1977): Diet quality in fish toxicology: Effects on acute and chronic toxicity. In: *Aquatic Toxicology and Hazard Evaluation*, edited by F. L. Mayer and J. L. Hamelink, pp. 269–280. American Society for Testing and Materials.
132. Melancon, M. J., and Lech, J. J. (1976a): Isolation and identification of a polar metabolite of tetrachlorobiphenyl from bile of rainbow trout exposed to ¹⁴C-tetrachlorobiphenyl. *Bull. Environ. Contam. Toxicol.*, 15:181–188.
133. Melancon, M. J., and Lech, J. J. (1976b): Distribution and biliary excretion products of di-2-ethylhexyl phthalate in rainbow trout. *Drug Metab. Dispos.*, 4:112–118.
134. Meyers, J. D. (1950): Net splanchnic glucose production in normal men and in various disease states. *J. Clin. Invest.*, 29:1,421–1,428.
135. Mount, D. I. (1962): Chronic effects of endrin on bluntnose minnows and guppies. *U.S. Fish Wildl. Serv., Res. Rep. 58.*

136. Mukherjie, S., and Bhattacharya, S. (1975): Histopathological lesions in the hepatopancreases of fishes exposed to industrial pollutants. *Indian J. Exp. Bio.*, 13:571–573.

137. Murdaugh, H. V., Robin, E. D., Millen, J. E., and Drewry, W. F. (1965): Cardiac output determination by the dye dilution method in *Squalus acanthius*. *Am. J. Physiol.*, 209:723–726.

138. Nestel, H., and Budd, J. (1975): Chronic oral exposure of rainbow trout (*Salmo gairdneri*) to a polychlorinated biphenyl (Aroclor 1254): Pathological effects. *Can. J. Comp. Med.*, 33:208–215.

139. Neutz, J. M., Wyler, F., and Rudolf, A. M. (1968): Changes in distribution of cardiac output after hemorrhage in rabbits. *Am. J. Physiol.*, 215:857–864.

140. Nopanitaya, W., Carson, J. L., Grisham, J. W., and Aghajanian, J. G. (1979): New observations on the fine structure of the liver in goldfish (*Carassius auratus*). *Cell Tissue Res.*, 196:249–261.

141. Novikoff, A. B. (1964): Cell heterogeneity within the hepatic lobule of the rat (staining reaction). *J. Histochem. Cytochem.*, 7:240–244.

142. Ochiai, A., Umeda, S., and Ogawa, M. (1974): On the acceleration of maturity of the catadromous female eel by hormone injection, and changes in the liver and blood character. *Bull. Jap. Soc. Sci. Fish.*, 40:43–50.

143. Oguri, M. (1978): Histochemical observations on the interrenal gland and liver of European spotted dogfish. *Bull. Jap. Soc. Sci. Fish.*, 44:703–707.

144. Peute, J., van der Gaag, M. A., Lambert, J. G. D. (1978): Ultrastructure and lipid content of the zebrafish *Branchydanio rerio* related to vitellogin synthesis. *Cell Tissue Res.*, 186:297–308.

145. Pfeifer, K. F. (1978): *Biochemical and physiological aspects of carbon tetrachloride (CCl₄) toxicity in the rainbow trout (Salmo gairdneri).* Ph.D Thesis, Oregon State University, Corvallis.

146. Pfeifer, K. F., and Weber, L. J. (1979): The effect of carbon tetrachloride on the total plasma protein concentration of rainbow trout (*Salmo gairdneri*). *Comp. Biochem. Physiol.*,64:37–42.

147. Pfeifer, K. F., and Weber, L. J. (1980): The effect of carbon tetrachloride treatment on urine flow rate of the rainbow trout (*Salmo gairdneri*). *Toxicol. Appl. Pharmacol.*, 52:347–350.

148. Pfeifer, K. F., Weber, L. J., and Larson, R. E. (1977): Alanine aminotransferase (GPT) in rainbow trout: Plasma enzyme levels as an index of liver damage. *Proc. West Pharmacol. Soc.*, 20:431–437.

149. Pfeifer, K. F., Weber, L. J., and Larson, R. E. (1980): Carbon tetrachloride-induced hepatotoxic response in rainbow trout, *Salmo gairdneri*, as influenced by two commercial fish diets. *Comp. Biochem. Physiol.*, 67C:91–96.

150. Plaa, G. L. (1968): Evaluation of liver function methodology. In: *Selected Pharmacological Testing Methods*, edited by Alfred Burger, pp. 255–288. Marcel Dekker, Inc. New York.

151. Rabinovici, N., and Wiener, E. (1963): Hemodynamic changes in the hepatectomized liver of the rat and their relationships to regeneration. *J. Surg. Res.*, 3:3–8.

152. Racicot, J. G., Gaudet, M., and Leray, C. (1975): Blood and liver enzymes in rainbow trout (*Salmo gairdneri* Rich.) with emphasis on their diagnostic use: Study with CCl₄ toxicity and a case of *Aeromonas* infection. *J. Fish Biol.*, 7:825–835.

153. Rappaport, A. M. (1975): Anatomic considerations. In: *Diseases of the Liver*, edited by L. Schiff, pp. 1–50. J. B. Lippincott, Philadelphia.

154. Redinger, R. N., Hermann, A. H., and Small, D. M. (1973): Primate biliary physiology: X. Effects of diet and fasting on biliary lipid secretion and relative composition of bile salt metabolism in rhesus monkey. *Gastroenterology*, 64:610–621.

155. Roberts, R. J. (1978): The anatomy and physiology of teleosts. In: *Fish Pathology*, edited by R. J. Roberts, pp. 13–54. Bailliere Tindall, London.

156. Sakaguchi, T. T., and Hamaguchi, A. (1975): Physiological changes in the serum and hepatopancreas of yellowtail injected with carbon tetrachloride. *Bull. Jap. Soc. Sci. Fish.*, 41:283–390.

157. Sastry, K. V., and Agrawal, V. P. (1976): Histochemical studies on the liver of *Heteropneustes fossilis* treated with carbon tetrachloride. *Acta Anat.*, 94:59–64.

158. Sastry, K. V., Agrawal, V. P., and Garg, V. K. (1976): Distribution of glucose-6-phosphatase and 5-nucleotidase in the digestive system of two teleost fishes. *Acta Histochem.*, 57:183–190.

159. Sastry, K. V., and Sharma, S. K. (1978): The effect of endrin on the histopathological changes in the liver of *Channa punctatus*. *Bull Environ. Contam. Toxicol.*, 20:674–677.

160. Satchell, G. H. (1971): *Circulation in Fishes*. Cambridge University Press, New York.

161. Sauer, D. M., and Haider, G. (1977): Enzyme activities in the serum of rainbow trout, *Salmo gairdneri* Richardson; The effects of water temperature. *J. Fish Biol.*, 11:605–612.

162. Scarpelli, D. G., Greider, M. H., and Frajola, W. J. (1963): Observations on hepatic cell hyperplasia, adenoma, and hepatoma of rainbow trout (*Salmo gairdneri*). *Cancer Res.*, 23:848–857.

163. Schmidt, D. C., and Weber, L. J. (1973): Metabolism and biliary excretion of sulfobromophthalein by rainbow trout. *J. Fish. Res. Board Can.*, 30:1,301–1,308.

164. Schoenhard, G. L., Lee, D. J., Howell, S. E., Pawlowski, N. E., Libbey. L. M., and Sinnhuber, R. O. (1976): Aflatoxin B₁ metabolism to aflatoxicol and derivatives lethal to *Bacillus subtilis* GSY 1057 by rainbow trout (*Salmo gairdneri*) liver. *Cancer Res.*, 36:2,040–2,045.

165. Schoor, W. P., and Couch, J. A. (1979): Correlation of mixed function oxidase activity with ultrastructural changes in the liver of a marine fish. *Cancer Biochem. Biophys.*, 4:95–103.

166. Seawright, A. A., and McLean, A. E. M. (1967): The effect of diet on carbon tetrachloride metabolism. *Biochem. J.*, 105:1,055–1,060.

167. Shank, R. E., Morrison, C. E., Changi, C. H. H., Karl, J., and Schwartz, D. R. (1959): Cell heterogeneity within the hepatic lobule (quantitative histochemistry). *J. Histochem. Cytochem.*, 7:237–244.
168. Shin, Y. C. (1977): Some observations on the fine structure of lamprey liver as revealed by electron microscopy. *Okajimas Folia Anat. Jap.*, 54:25–60.
169. Simon, R. C., Dollar, A. M., and Smuckler, E. A. (1967): Descriptive classification on normal and altered histology of trout livers. In: *Trout Hepatoma Research Conference Papers*, edited by J. E. Halver and I. A. Mitchell, pp. 18–28. *U.S. Fish Wildl. Serv., Res. Rep. 70.*
170. Sinclair, D. A. R., and Eales, J. G. (1972): Iodothyroxine-glucuronide conjugates in the bile of brook trout, *Salvelinus fontinalis* (Mitchill) and other freshwater teleosts. *Gen. Comp. Endocrinol.*, 19:552–559.
171. Sorensen, E. M. B. (1976): Ultrastructural changes in the hepatocytes of green sunfish, *Lepomis cyanellus* Rafinesque, exposed to solution of sodium arsenate. *J. Fish Biol.*, 8:229–240.
172. Statham, C. N., Croft, W. A., and Lech, J. J. (1978): Uptake, distribution, and effects of carbon tetrachloride in rainbow trout (*Salmo gairdneri*). *Toxicol. Appl. Pharmacol.*, 45:131–140.
173. Statham, C. N., Melancon, M. J., Jr., and Lech, J. J. (1976): Bioconcentration of xenobiotics in trout bile: A proposed monitoring aid for some waterborne chemicals. *Science*, 193:680–681.
174. Stevens, E. D. (1968): The effect of exercise on the distribution of blood to various organs in rainbow trout. *Comp. Biochem. Physiol.*, 25:614–625.
175. Stott, W. T., and Sinnhuber, R. O. (1978): Dietary casein levels and aflatoxin B$_1$ metabolism in rainbow trout (*Salmo gairdneri*). In: *Pesticide and Xenobiotic Metabolism in Aquatic Organisms*, edited by M. A. Q. Khan, J. J. Lech, and J. J. Menn, pp. 389–400. ACS Symposium Series 99, American Chemical Society, Washington, DC.
176. Swallow, R. L., and Fleming, W. R. (1969): The effect of starvation, feeding, glucose, and ACTH on the liver glycogen levels of *Tilapia mossambica*. *Comp. Biochem. Physiol.*, 28:95–106.
177. Thilenius, O. G., Hoffer, P. B., Fitzgerald, R. S., and Perkins, J. F. (1963): Response of pulmonary circulation of resting, unanesthetized dogs to acute hypoxia. *Am. J. Physiol.*, 206:867–874.
178. Truscott, B. (1979): Steroid metabolism in fish. Identification of steroid moieties of hydrolyzable conjugates of cortisol in the bile of trout, *Salmo gairdneri*. *Gen. Comp. Endocrinol.*, 38:196–206.
179. Truscott, B., Kane, K. M., and Idler, D. R. (1978): 21-Hydroxy-pregna-1,4-diene-3,11,20-trione: A biliary metabolite of a cartilaginous fish, *Raja* sp. *Steroids*, 31:573–582.
180. Tucker, R. K., and Leitzke, J. S. (1979): Comparative toxicology of insecticides for vertebrate wildlife and fish. *J. Pharmacol. Ther.*, 6:167–220.
181. Vernier, J. M. (1974): Ultrastructural studies of very low density hepatic lipoproteins during the development of the rainbow trout (*Salmo gairdneri*). *J. Microscopie Biol. Cell.*, 23:39–50.

182. Weinreb, E. L., and Bilstad, N. M. (1955): Histology of the digestive tract and adjacent structures of the rainbow trout *Salmo gairdneri irideus*. *Copeia*, 1955:194–204.
183. Weis, P. (1972): Hepatic ultrastructure in two species of normal, fasted, and gravid teleost fishes. *Am. J. Anat.*, 133:317–332.
184. Weis, P. (1974): Ultrastructural changes induced by low concentrations of DDT in the livers of zebrafish and guppy. *Chem.-Biol. Interact.*, 8:25–30.
185. Welsch, U. N., and Storch, V. W. (1973): Enzyme histochemical and ultrastructural observations on the liver of teleost fishes. *Arch. Histol. Jap.*, 36:21–37.
186. White, S. W., Chalmers, J. P., and Hilder, R. (1967): Local thermodilution method for measuring blood flow in the portal and renal veins of the unanesthetized rabbit. *Aust. J. Exp. Biol. Med. Sci.*, 45:453.
187. Witte, C. L., and Witte, M. H. (1974): Hepatic circulation. In: *The Liver: Normal and Abnormal Functions. Part A*, edited by F. F. Becker, pp. 12–54. Marcel Dekker, Inc., New York.
188. Wodtke, E. (1978): Lipid adaptation in liver mitochondrial membranes of carp acclimated to different environmental temperatures. *Biochim. Biophys. Acta*, 529:280–291.
189. Yamamoto, T. (1965): Some observations on the fine structure of the intrahepatic biliary passages in goldfish (*Carassius auratus*). *Z. Zellforsch. Mikrosk. Anat.*, 65:319–330.
190. Yarbrough, J. D., and Chambers, J. E. (1977): Crude oil effects on microsomal mixed-function oxidase system components in the striped mullet (*Mugil cephalus*). *Life Sci.*, 21:1,095–1,100.
191. Yarbrough, J. D., Neitz, J. R., and Chambers, J. O. (1976): Physiological effects of crude oil exposure in the striped mullet *Mugil cephalus*. *Life Sci.*, 19:775–780.

*Aquatic Toxicology*, edited by Lavern J. Weber,
Raven Press, New York © 1982.

# Induction of Monooxygenase Activity in Fish

John J. Lech, Mary Jo Vodicnik, and
*C. R. Elcombe

*Department of Pharmacology and Toxicology, The Medical College of
Wisconsin, Milwaukee, Wisconsin 53226; and The Great Lakes Research
Facility, University of Wisconsin, Milwaukee, Wisconsin 53201,
*Central Toxicology Laboratory, Imperial Chemical Industries,
Macclesfield, Cheshire, England*

Although the oxidation and conjugation of drugs and xenobiotic chemicals in mammals have been extensively studied in the past, it is only in recent years that attention has been devoted to these phenomena in aquatic species. Catalyzed by a critical need for knowledge concerning the persistence and fate of chemicals in fish and other aquatic species, significant advances in this field have been made of late. It has been firmly established over the past ten years that fish are able to oxidize and conjugate many foreign chemicals, and the biochemical systems responsible for these oxidations and conjugations are qualitatively, if not quantitatively, similar to those found in mammals and avian species (1,13,19,35). Much of the early work concerning biotransformation systems in fish and other aquatic species was performed *in vitro* and was largely patterned after early studies done with tissue fractions from a variety of mammalian species. A progression from *in vitro* studies to *in vivo* investigations in recent years has provided evidence that biotransformation of many xenobiotic chemicals occurs in the intact fish and that these processes may lead to the formation of more toxic materials, as well as less biologically active products (53,72).

Since oxidation, conjugation, and hydrolysis are major determinants of the fate, persistence, and toxicity of drugs and chemicals,

the importance of changes in the activity of the biological systems
responsible for these processes was quickly recognized; the phenomenon of induction of monooxygenase (MO) activity has been
intensively studied and reviewed over the past 20 years (23,85,102).
In the face of much available information concerning the induction
of MOs by xenobiotic chemicals in mammalian and avian species,
literature concerning this phenomenon in fish has only begun to
appear in the last few years. However, this is not surprising when
the rather slow development of concepts concerning biotransformation systems in aquatic species is considered. The reasons for the
recent expansion of interest in induction phenomena in fish range
from the practical consideration concerning the use of hepatic MO
in aquatic species for environmental monitoring to academic questions concerning comparative aspects of the modulation of these
systems in lower life forms.

## INDUCTION OF CYTOCHROME(S) P-450 AND MONOOXYGENASE ACTIVITY IN FISH

### The MO System

The oxidation of many xenobiotic chemicals is catalyzed by a
group of hepatic, internal MOs, which require the cofactor NADPH
and molecular oxygen for the oxidative process. While hydroxylation of certain compounds in mammalian liver has been demonstrated to be due to a flavoprotein oxidase, much of the oxidative
activity in liver has been shown to reside in enzyme systems (MO)
comprised of carbon monoxide-sensitive oxidases known as cyto-
chrome(s) P-450 and a flavoprotein, NADPH-cytochrome P-450
reductase. The MO system in mammalian liver has been demonstrated by tissue fractionation and marker enzyme techniques to
reside primarily in the smooth endoplasmic reticulum, and is characterized by a relatively low degree of substrate specificity when
compared to enzymes of intermediary metabolism. In general terms,
the MO system has been shown to catalyze a variety of reactions,
including aromatic and aliphatic N-hydroxylation, N-dealkylation,

and o-dealkylation. The general scheme for these reactions is shown in Fig. 1A; it can be seen that molecular oxygen can either be incorporated into the parent compound or the leaving alkyl group (Fig. 1B and C). For the sake of simplicity, the intermediate steps in these reactions are not shown.

Numerous substrates have been used to study MO activity *in vitro*, and many of these are drugs and chemicals which are known to be oxidized by hepatic MO systems *in vivo*. Thus, positive or negative alterations of MO activity in liver fractions have been assayed using aniline (aniline hydroxylase), para-nitroanisole, (para-nitroanisole-o-demethylase), aminopyrine (aminopyrine-N-demethylase), ethylmorphine (ethylmorphine-N-demethylase), and benzo(a)pyrene (aromatic hydrocarbonhydroxylase, AHH). These enzyme activities have been repeatedly studied in many mammalian and avian species and have recently been demonstrated in many species of fish (35,63,92). It should be recognized at this point that although the generic term "fish" will be used throughout this chapter, the term is used loosely, and it is to be expected that activities of these enzymes among fish species will be as varied quantitatively as they are among mammalian species.

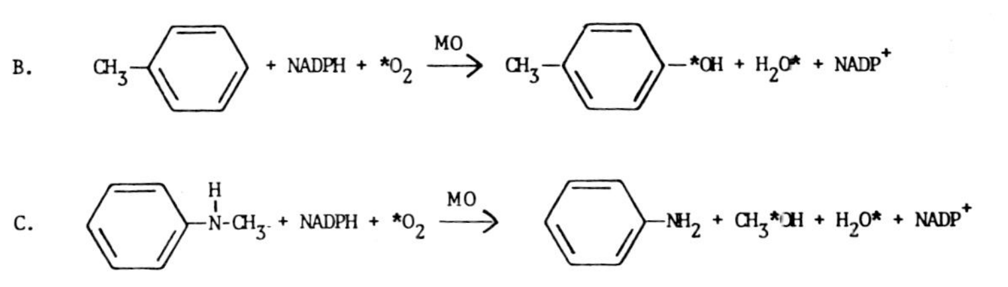

FIG. 1. **A:** Scheme of the hepatic microsomal P-450 MO system. **B** and **C:** Examples of oxidations catalyzed by MOs.

Several lines of evidence from the mammalian literature have indicated that there is a certain degree of specificity for classes of xenobiotic chemicals as substrates among the MO systems in mammals, and this specificity is thought to be conferred by multiple forms of cytochrome(s) P-450, the terminal oxidase in MO systems (76,85,102). Although it has been known for some time that two types of CO-binding cytochromes exist in mammalian liver microsomes, cytochrome P-450 and cytochrome P-448, at least six forms have been recently described (50,56,115).

It should be noted that cytochrome P-448 was initially described and differentiated from cytochrome P-450 through the use of chemical inducers of the MO system. The microsomal cytochromes are nominally characterized by the absorption maximum wavelength ($\lambda$ max) of their reduced CO difference spectra. Spectral changes including the appearance of a $\lambda$max of 448 nm rather than 450 nm in microsomes from 3-methylcholanthrene- (3-MC) pretreated animals, along with increased MO activity, were evidence that pointed towards the induction of cytochrome P-448 (9,101). The classic MO inducer, phenobarbital, increases MO activity and cytochrome P-450 levels, but the $\lambda$max of the CO difference spectra of reduced microsomes remains at 450 nm.

These early observations with 3-MC and phenobarbital have led to the concept of two major classes of MO-inducing chemicals, and these classes have been traditionally known as 3-MC-like and phenobarbital-like, although the existence of atypical inducers such as caffeine, ethanol, pregnenolone-16$\alpha$-carbonitrile (PCN), and safrole has been demonstrated (102). These broad classes of inducers have been defined largely through the spectrum of enzymes that are induced (substrate specificity), the spectral properties and electrophoretic patterns of induced cytochromes, and, more recently, by the immunochemical properties of the cytochromes themselves.

## MO Substrate Specificity

In order to understand and study the induction of cytochrome(s) P-450 and associated MOs in fish, it is important to recognize the characteristics of the substrates that have been used in mammalian MO assays and the properties of cytochrome(s) P-450 in mammalian systems. Table 1 lists commonly used substrates in studies of MO systems in mammalian liver microsomes and the responses of these activities to 3-MC-like and phenobarbital-like inducing agents. While activities 3 through 7 are increased by both classes of inducers and the response may vary in magnitude with species and strain of animal, 1 and 2 appear to be specific for phenobarbital-type induction and 8 appears to be specific for 3-MC-like induction. From the information in this table, it is apparent that studies of MO systems in fish must utilize substrates that will indicate the type of induction produced by a given chemical agent. For example, if AHH is increased by a particular inducing agent, it would be difficult to characterize the type of induction elicited, since AHH activity is enhanced by both phenobarbital-like and 3-MC-like inducers. On the other hand, some degree of specificity of the type of induction observed would be indicated by the use of benzphetamine-N-demethylase (BeND) or ethoxyresorufin-o-deethylase (EROD) activities (17,76).

TABLE 1. *Responses of mammalian liver MO[a] activities to phenobarbital and 3-MC*

|  | Phenobarbital induction | 3-MC induction |
|---|---|---|
| 1. BeND | +[b] | −[c] |
| 2. Ethylmorphine-N-demethylase | + | − |
| 3. Aniline hydroxylase | + | + |
| 4. p-nitroanisole-o-demethylase | + | + |
| 5. Aminopyrine-N-demethylase | + | + |
| 6. AHH | + | + |
| 7. ECOD | + | + |
| 8. EROD | − | + |

[a]MO = Monooxygenase.
[b]+ = Increase in activity.
[c]− = No change or decrease.
Constructed from ref. 17,23,24,64,77,116,119.

Although the MO activities noted in Table 1 have been reported to occur in fish liver (13,35) and several have been shown to increase with polycyclic aromatic hydrocarbon inducers, few studies have analyzed the response of fish liver MOs with a spectrum of assays of suitable breadth to characterize the nature of induction. Although specific inducers will be discussed in later sections, polycyclic aromatic hydrocarbons appear to induce a pattern of MO activities in the rainbow trout (*Salmo gairdneri*) (38) and in the sheepshead (*Archosargus probatocephalus*) (61) that resembles that of 3-MC in rats and other mammals. On the other hand, the response of fish liver MO to phenobarbital-type inducers, be they drugs or xenobiotic chemicals, has not been clearly demonstrated, and few attempts have been made to address this point through the use of multiple MO substrates. Although evidence will be presented later to illustrate that several species of fish do not respond to phenobarbital-type inducers, it should be noted at this point that studies of the MO system in fish cannot proceed rationally without using, as a reference point, common assay systems and criteria that have been established for the MO system in mammals.

## Cytochrome(s) P-450 in Fish

In view of the facts that the identifiable forms of cytochrome(s) P-450 in mammalian liver have risen from two to at least six and that the classification of inducers as 3-MC-like or phenobarbital-like has been challenged by the appearance of atypical inducers, it is important to define certain terms for purposes of discussion in order to avoid confusion with the current literature. In a recent review, Nebert (85) has defined cytochrome(s) P-450 as all forms of membrane-bound hemoprotein associated with NADPH-dependent MO activities and capable of binding CO when reduced. Cytochrome $P_1$-450 was defined as the polycyclic aromatic hydrocarbon-inducible form(s) of cytochrome(s) P-450 associated with induced AHH activity; and cytochrome P-448 was defined as the polycyclic aromatic hydrocarbon-inducible form of cytochrome(s) P-450 associated with the greatest hypsochromic (blue) shift in the $\lambda$max of the Soret peak of the reduced hemoprotein-CO complex. From these definitions it would appear that spectral as well as appropriate enzymatic assays must be carried out in induction studies with polycyclic aromatic hydrocarbons in order to differentiate between the inducible forms of cytochrome $P_1$-450. Further characterization of induced cytochrome(s) P-450 has been done by the use of sodium dodecyl sulfate-polyacrylamide gel electrophoresis (SDS-PAGE), with appropriate staining for protein and heme and subsequent determination of the apparent molecular weight of the new or enhanced hemoprotein bands (10,125). In addition, hepatic cytochrome(s) P-450 from mammals have been solubilized and purified by chromatographic techniques and characterized spectrally, enzymatically, and immunologically (50,76,115). The specific terminologies (57) for these cytochromes will not be introduced here, since few, if any, studies using fish have progressed to an advanced stage in which an in-depth discussion would be appropriate or meaningful. Table 2 illustrates some properties and levels of hepatic cytochrome(s) P-450 that have been described in both control and "induced" fish. While more exhaustive compilations of cytochrome(s) P-450 levels in fish are given elsewhere (4,13,103), several important pieces of information are illustrated. In general, the Soret λmax in most species studied occurs at approximately 450 nm, and there is no spectral shift observable in the induced state. This observation has been reported by several investigators, even when induction of MO activities by polycyclic aromatic hydrocarbon inducers was as high as 20- to 40-fold (22,38,45,90). It has been reported, however, that CO-ligated reduced microsomes from livers of 3-MC-pretreated scup (*Stenotomus versicolor*) had an absorption λmax at 448 nm (112) as did microsomes from 3-MC-pretreated sheepshead (61), but the reasons for this have not been fully explored. Type I and Type II binding spectra similar to those described for mammalian cytochrome(s) P-450 have been observed in several investigations (24,30,33) and the ethylisocyanide (ETNC) peak ratios, often used to distinguish between different forms of cytochrome(s) P-450 in mammals, shift to higher values in β naphthoflavone (βNF)-induced rainbow trout (38). It has been reported that

TABLE 2. Concentrations and properties of hepatic microsomal cytochrome(s) P-450 in several species of fish

| Species | Specific content (pmole/mg microsomal prot) | CO Spectra λmax (nm) | Type I substrate binding | Type II substrate binding | ETNC 455/430 | Ref. |
|---|---|---|---|---|---|---|
| *Salmo trutta* | | | | | | |
| Control | 396 | 450.6 | ± | + | 0.35 | 6 |
| *Salmo gairdneri* | | | | | | |
| Control | 234 | 449 | + | + | 0.28 | 38 |
| Treated[a] | 341 | 449 | − | − | 0.44 | |
| *Stenotomus versicolor* | | | | | | |
| Control | 620 | 450 | − | − | — | 109 |
| *Salmo gairdneri* | | | | | | |
| Control | 210 | 450 | − | − | — | 73 |
| Treated[b] | 320 | — | − | − | — | 73 |
| *Ictalurus punctatus* | | | | | | |
| Control | 237 | 450 | − | − | — | 18 |
| Treated[c] | 702 | — | − | − | — | |
| *Fundulus heteroclitus* | | | | | | |
| Control | 9 | 450 | − | − | — | 18 |
| Treated[d] | 97 | — | − | − | — | |
| *Archosargus probatocephalus* | | | | | | |
| Control | 280 | 450 | − | − | — | 13 |
| Treated[e] | 280 | — | − | − | — | |

[a] βNF—100 mg/kg (i.p.), sacrificed at 4 days.
[b] Clophen A50—1 g/kg by mouth, sacrificed at 7 days.
[c] Aroclor 1254—50 mg/kg (i.p.), daily for 7 days.
[d] Phenylbutazone—100 μg/l in seawater, 10 days.
[e] Phenylbutazone—20 mg/kg (i.p.), on days 1 and 3, sacrificed day 6.

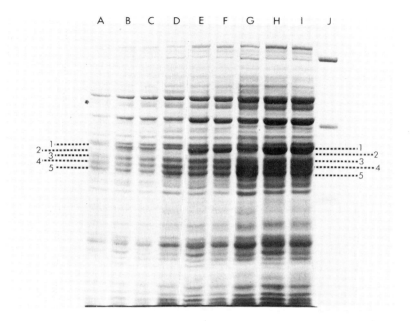

**FIG. 2.** SDS-PAGE of hepatic microsomes from rainbow trout pretreated with various inducers. **A, D,** and **G:** Control (corn oil) microsomes at loadings of 45, 90, and 180 μg protein. **B, E,** and **H:** β-NF microsomes (100 mg/kg) at loadings as above. Bands 1, 2, 3, 4, and 5 correspond to 59,500; 57,000; 51,000; 48,000; and 45,000 daltons respectively. (From Elcombe and Lech, ref. 38.)

in uninduced rainbow trout, the pH dependency of the ETNC-cytochrome(s) P-450 interaction spectral peaks is similar to that of control rats, rather than that from 3-MC-treated rats (4,90).

Data are also shown in Table 2 for control and phenylbutazone-treated fish (*Fundulus heteroclitus* and sheepshead) to illustrate discrepancies that have been reported with the use of phenobarbital-type inducers in fish. It is not known if the induction observed in *Fundulus* is related to a species or treatment protocol difference, but evidence which will be discussed later indicates that the responses to phenobarbital-type inducers in fish are not typical of their inductive effect in mammals (2,11,13,16,38,52,97).

It is clear that most species of fish studied respond well to 3-MC-type inducers and that the MO activities that are increased are the specific and nonspecific indicators of this type of induction in mammals. Likewise, it has also been shown that MO activities characteristic of phenobarbital-type inducers are not increased under conditions in which maximal induction of MO enzymes associated with 3-MC-type induction is observed (36,38).

SDS-PAGE of microsomes from variously induced rats has been used to attempt to characterize cytochrome(s) P-450 by banding patterns and apparent molecular weights (10,125). Although molecular weights of cytochrome(s) P-450 may differ when intact microsomes are compared to purified cytochromes, characteristic cytochrome "patterns" have been recognized with various types of inducers. SDS-PAGE of solubilized rainbow trout liver microsomes showed several Coomassie blue- and peroxidase-staining bands in the 40,000 to 60,000 dalton region (Fig. 2). Microsomes from βNF-induced rainbow trout exhibited an enhanced band(s) at 57,000 daltons when compared to microsomes from control fish (24). The pattern seen closely resembled that seen in rats treated with βNF, except that in rats, the band appeared in the 53,000 dalton region using the same SDS-PAGE system. Although the band that appeared in microsomes from βNF-treated trout stained both for the heme and protein, there is no direct proof that the intensification of this band was causally related to the increased MO activities observed.

While it is not possible to generalize among all species of fish, several lines of evidence indicate that the 3-MC-type inducers elevate cytochrome(s) P-450 in liver and are best termed cytochrome(s) $P_1$-450 according to the definitions cited earlier. The spectrum of MO activities induced, the ETNC peak ratios, the Soret λmax, the SDS-PAGE banding, and the behavior of the induced MO activities towards *in vitro* inhibition by α-naphthoflavone (α-NF) (4,13,38,109) are all characteristic of cytochrome $P_1$-450. The general absence of a hypsochromic shift in the Soret λmax in liver microsomes from induced fish is the major feature that does not allow the assignment of cytochrome P-448 at the present time. It is possible that several cytochrome(s) $P_1$-450 are induced, including cytochrome P-448, but the concentration of the latter in microsomes is not sufficient to permit the observation of an overall spectral shift due to the presence of much higher concentrations of cytochrome(s) P-450 that have their $\lambda$max at control wavelengths. There is evidence to suggest that this explanation is plausible, since a cytochrome from 1,2,3,4,-dibenzanthrene-induced little skate (*Raja erinacea*) has been partially purified and was shown to have a $\lambda$max at 448 nm, even though there was no difference in $\lambda$max (450 nm) between intact microsomes from control and induced animals (12).

## Factors Affecting Induction

From the data presented in the preceding section, it should be obvious that certain classes of compounds, notably 3-MC-like inducers, are able to produce a phenomenon in fish that is similar to induction of MO in mammals. However, the use of the word induction implies *de novo* synthesis of cytochrome(s) P-450 and should be clearly distinguished from activation of MO activity. Studies done in the past with phenobarbital- and 3-MC-type inducers have established that these compounds are inducers of MO, not merely activators (24,25,44). Induction is characterized by a relatively long latent period after pretreatment with a chemical (approximately 2 to 4 days) for the appearance of increased levels of cytochrome(s) P-450 or MO activity, and these increases can be blocked by pretreatment of the animals with inhibitors of protein synthesis such as puromycin (44) or actinomycin D (25,44). On the other hand, activation of nascent MO activity should be differentiated from induction and has been demonstrated *in vitro* by preincubation of several classes of compounds (including 3,4,-benzo[a]pyrene) with hepatic microsomes prior to assay of biphenyl 2-hydroxylase activity (78).

While investigations have differentiated induction from activation using MO systems from mammals, there have been few reports in the literature that have addressed whether or not the induction process observed in fish is truly a result of *de novo* synthesis of cytochrome(s) P-450, nor have there been any descriptions of activation of MO activity in fish hepatic microsomes *in vitro* (40). While there is no real reason to suspect that true inducers in mammals are not true inducers in fish, these classic mammalian experiments have not been, but should be, done to verify the induction phenomenon in fish.

In addition to these very basic experiments not yet performed, there is a litany of other variables that remain to be considered before the toxicological significance of induction of MO in fish by xenobiotic chemicals can be assessed. It is apparent that induction of cytochrome(s) P-450 and MO activity in fish by inducers of the phenobarbital class has not been clearly demonstrated. This is a very basic question; it must be established whether fish in general are not responsive to phenobarbital-type inducers or whether the negative data produced in past experiments with fish may have been related to experimental variables such as route and frequency of administration; absorption, distribution, and elimination of the inducer; age and sex of the fish used; environmental temperature; photoperiod; and pretreatment time course. These variables are almost certain to affect responses in fish to MO inducers. Several studies have demonstrated an influence of temperature, age, sex, and season on MO systems in fish and their response to several inducers (61,108,110).

In most reports concerning induction in fish, attention has been focused on levels of cytochrome(s) P-450 and MO activities, and only a few studies have been directed towards other components of the microsomal electron transport system. Small increases in the activity of NADPH cytochrome c reductase have been reported in hepatic microsomes from channel catfish (*Ictalurus punctatus*) treated with Aroclor 1254 (69); on the other hand, the PCB mixture Clophen A-50 failed to elevate this enzyme in hepatic microsomes of rainbow trout even though o-demethylation of *p*-nitroanisole and cytochrome(s) P-450 content were increased (42). While NADPH and NADH cytochrome c reductase as well as hexose-6-phosphate dehydrogenase in hepatic microsomal hydroxylations in fish have been studied (20,111), it is not known if any of the effects of inducers on MO activity can be attributed to actions at site(s) prior to the terminal oxidase cytochrome(s) P-450. It has been suggested that cytochrome(s) P-450 in trout microsomes may not be rate-limiting under certain circumstances (21,73). These other steps in the process of oxidation warrant further study with respect to inducers.

## DRUGS AND HORMONES

### Phenobarbital and Phenylbutazone

While in recent years, polycyclic aromatic hydrocarbons and halogenated hydrocarbons have been the classes of compounds most actively studied with regard to induction of MO in fish, drugs such as phenobarbital and phenylbutazone were the earliest compounds to be studied. Although phenobarbital is of less interest to environmental concerns than it is to academic interests within the area of MO induction, it will be discussed here largely because it has earned "prototype status" as an inducing agent, and because of its uncertain status as an inducer of MO in fish. Phenobarbital produces a type of MO induction in mammalian liver characterized by an increase in cytochrome(s) P-450 content without a change in λmax and a significant elevation of the MO activities illustrated in Table 1. It should be emphasized that while some of the enzyme activities listed in Table 1, such as AHH, can be elevated by phenobarbital- as well as 3-MC-type inducers, certain MO activities, including ethylmorphine-N-demethylase and BeND, are specific to phenobarbital-type induction. There are only a few studies in the literature that have reported the effects of phenobarbital and a related inducer, phenylbutazone, in fish, and, with one exception, these studies have failed to demonstrate significant induction of MO in the species studied. When *Fundulus heteroclitus* were exposed to 10 and 100 parts per billion of phenylbutazone in sea water for 10 days, hepatic microsomal cytochrome(s) P-450 levels rose 3- and 10-fold respectively, and *in vitro* rates of aldrin epoxidation were doubled and tripled (18). While other studies utilizing several species of fish deviated in experimental protocol from the work described with *Fundulus*, in terms of route of administration and pretreatment time course, they nevertheless failed to demonstrate significant induction of MO activities by this class of inducer (11,13,16,38,52). Several aspects of the response in *Fundulus* seem noteworthy. First, the control concentrations of cytochrome(s) P-450 were among the lowest reported in fish (controls had less than 9 pmole per mg of microsomal protein, Table 2), and the response to phenylbutazone was a 10-fold increase in cytochrome(s) P-450 content, which is the largest increase ever reported in fish. Since the low concentration of cytochrome(s) P-450 in control animals and the magnitude of the response to phenylbutazone were unusual, these experiments warrant further consideration to validate this observation with phenylbutazone in *Fundulus* and its relevance to other species of fish.

Other xenobiotic chemicals that have been shown to be phenobarbital-type inducers in rodents, such as DDT and noncoplanar polychlorinated biphenyl (PCB) isomers have proven to be ineffective as inducers in the species of fish given mammalian doses by the i.p. route (2,36). The reason for the lack of an inductive effect of phenobarbital-type inducers should be investigated more fully since, if refractivity to this class of inducer proves to be universal among fish, a knowledge of the basis for refractivity may be important in understanding the process of induction in higher life forms. Future studies with phenobarbital-type inducers should include a careful consideration of the pharmacokinetics and distribution of the inducing agents, the time course of pretreatment to observe induction, the route of administration, and the basal or control state of MO enzymes that are most likely to specifically reflect phenobarbital-type induction.

## Steroids

### Sex Steroids

It has been known for many years that male rats metabolize a number of drugs more rapidly than females; sex differences in the rate of drug metabolism have been demonstrated in a number of mammalian species. These differences in MO activity appear to be due, at least in part, to the action of sex steroid hormones (66).

Early studies in fish failed to demonstrate a sex-related difference in hepatic drug metabolism, possibly because of small sample sizes, substantial intraspecies variability, and/or the time of the reproductive cycle in which the investigations were carried out (16,35). More recently, it has been shown that male rainbow and brook (*Salvelinus fontinalis*) trout have significantly higher hepatic microsomal cytochrome(s) P-450 content and aminopyrine demethylase activity than females during the spawning season, although a sex difference was not observed in the activity of the NADPH-linked electron transport system as measured by NADPH cytochrome c reductase activity (106,110). Cytochrome(s) P-450 content was also reported to be greater in kidney microsomes from male fish when compared to females. There was, in addition, a pronounced difference between sexes in the response of hepatic microsomal AHH activity to $\alpha$NF *in vitro*, suggesting the presence of different form(s) of cytochrome(s) P-450 in males and females. These differences were not demonstrable in gonadally immature animals, but whether sex steroids were involved in these phenomena, as is the case in the mammalian system, remains to be determined.

Preliminary data indicated that fish respond to inducers of MO activity differently, depending on their reproductive condition at the time of exposure (123). There is evidence that basal, hepatic microsomal AHH activity and its inducibility by petroleum exposure were suppressed in male and female cunners (*Tautogolabrus adspersus*) during the prespawning and spawning seasons, presumably when sex steroid levels are high, to promote spermatogenesis and vitellogenesis (123). Although the investigators did not consider a possible role of steroids in their observations, data are available that show that estradiol pretreatment of immature rainbow trout significantly reduced the magnitude of induction of hepatic MO activity by $\beta$NF in these animals as determined by cytochrome(s) P-450 content, and ethoxycoumarin-o-deethylation (ECOD) and EROD activities (*unpublished observations*). Although the significance of this observation is not known, it is interesting to note that various

MO activities are reduced during pregnancy in mammals (41) and that late-pregnant female rats become refractive to induction by cytochrome(s) P-450-type inducers, although their response to cytochrome(s) $P_1$-450-type inducers appears unaffected (51). It is postulated that this decrease in MO activity serves to ensure elevated steroid levels for the maintenance of pregnancy. While it is not possible to propose a common mechanism with respect to reproduction and MO activity in fish and mammals, the similarities noted are intriguing. Furthermore, the seasonal appearance of sex differences in prespawning and spawning fish suggests their use as models for studying the regulation of sex steroid-dependent form(s) of cytochrome(s) P-450.

### *Pregnenolone-16α-Carbonitrile (PCN)*

PCN is a synthetic progesterone derivative that has been shown to induce a cytochrome(s) P-450 profile in mammals that differs from that induced by phenobarbital with respect to substrate specificity, immunochemical properties, and electrophoretic mobility of the induced protein(s) (15,39,56,77,98).

It has been demonstrated that PCN administration to immature rainbow trout for 5 days at 25 mg/kg or 150 mg/kg resulted in a significant increase in the yield of hepatic microsomal protein, BeND, and ECOD activities without an effect on cytochrome(s) P-450 content or EROD (121). Since fish appear to be refractive to phenobarbital-type induction of MO activity, it is interesting to note that these activities characteristic of phenobarbital-type inducers were elevated in fish by PCN.

### *Adrenal Steroids*

In mammals, the adrenal gland is apparently necessary for the maintenance of normal, hepatic microsomal MO activity. Adrenalectomy results in a decrease in cytochrome(s) P-450 content in rats as well as an impairment of the metabolism of a number of substrates of the MO system, including steroid hormones. Whether an effect is observed on the NADPH-dependent electron transport system is, as yet, uncertain. In many cases, these effects on MO activity can be reversed by glucocorticoid administration (67). When cortisol pellets are implanted intraperitoneally into immature rainbow trout, a significant increase in NADPH cytochrome c reductase activity is observed, with no effect on microsomal cytochrome(s) P-450 or protein content (54). The investigators did not, however, measure microsomal MO activity. Elucidation of the role of glucocorticoids with respect to MO activity in fish is complicated by the fact that adrenal tissue, in most cases, is intermingled with kidney tissue, and thus, ablation of the "gland" is prohibited. At present, the influence of the adrenal gland in fish on MO activity remains enigmatic.

## POLYCYCLIC AROMATIC HYDROCARBONS

### 3-MC, Benzanthracene, and βNF

While phenobarbital-type inducers were probably the first class of inducing agents to be studied in fish, much attention has been focused in recent years on polycyclic aromatic hydrocarbon-type inducers. The effects of 3-MC on MO activity and cytochrome(s) P-450 content have been studied extensively in many species of mammals, and this compound has become somewhat of a standard against which many other polycyclic aromatic hydrocarbon inducers are compared. As mentioned, microsomes from mammals pretreated with 3-MC exhibit a characteristic pattern of induced MO activity (Table 1) which is different from control microsomes or microsomes prepared from phenobarbital-treated animals; the Soret λmax of the CO-difference spectra of reduced microsomes shifts from 450 to 448 nm.

The earliest and most frequently investigated polycyclic aromatic hydrocarbons in fish were 3-MC, benzanthracene, βNF, and, to some extent, benzo(a)pyrene. In the majority of cases, studies concerning the induction of hepatic MO activities in fish were limited to measurements of cytochrome(s) P-450 levels and only one or two selected MO activities that were inadequate to characterize the pattern of induction. Largely through an increasing interest in the ecological and toxicological effects of oil pollution, the number of polycyclic aromatic hydrocarbons studied for inductive effects in fish has been extended to include various crude oils and fractions thereof, and several pure components of oil, including pyrene, phenanthrene, fluoranthrene, chrysene, and dibenzothiophene. Table 2 illustrates the effects of a variety of polycyclic aromatic hydrocarbons that have been studied with respect to induction of cytochrome(s) P-450 and selected MO activities in fish. It can be seen that the most frequently studied MO activity was AHH; few studies have been concerned with the assay of other MO activities that have been used to characterize responses to polycyclic aromatic hydrocarbons in mammals. It is important to note that the data listed in Table 2 are compiled from a variety of literature sources and, in many cases, the failure to demonstrate induction may be related to species differences, the lack of dose-response curves, and comparable treatment periods among the experiments reported. It should also be noted that some studies have used the i.p. route of administration of these compounds, while others have used water exposure. In studies that were comprehensive enough to measure a spectrum of MO activities as well as cytochrome(s) P-450 content, it is clear that when specific polycyclic aromatic hydrocarbons are active as inducers, they appear to produce a pattern of induction of MO activities characteristic of 3-MC-type induction in mammals, and although cytochrome(s) P-450 levels are generally increased, there have been few reports of a shift in the Soret $\lambda$max to 448 nm. Although the magnitude of the increases in enzyme activities varies considerably and is probably species- and/or dose-related, AHH, aniline hydroxylase, ECOD, and EROD are typically elevated, while ethylmorphine-N-demethylase and BeND activities are usually unchanged or reduced (Table 3). Several experiments have been designed to attempt to characterize the cytochrome(s) P-450 induced in 1,2,3,4-dibenzanthracene-treated skates (13). Sodium cholate-

TABLE 3. *Effect of polycyclic aromatic hydrocarbons on cytochrome(s) P-450 content and various MO activities in fish*

| Inducer | Species | P-450 Content | AHH | AH[a] | ECOD | EROD | BeND | Reference |
|---|---|---|---|---|---|---|---|---|
| 3-MC | Sheepshead | —[b] | +[c] | ND | + | + | — | 97 |
| | Little skate | ND[d] | + | ND | + | + | + | 62 |
| | Southern flounder | — | + | ND | + | ND | — | 62 |
| | Atlantic stingray | — | + | ND | + | ND | — | 62 |
| | Brook trout | + | ND | + | + | ND | ND | 3 |
| | Scup | ND | + | ND | ND | ND | ND | 105 |
| | Steelhead trout | ND | + | ND | ND | ND | ND | 89 |
| | Rainbow trout | + | + | ND | + | + | — | 37,90,104 |
| | Northern pike | — | + | ND | ND | ND | ND | 11 |
| | Brown trout | + | + | ND | ND | ND | ND | 97 |
| | Carp | + | + | ND | — | + | — | 82 |
| 1,2,3,4-Dibenzanthracene | Sheepshead | — | + | ND | + | + | — | 61 |
| | Little skate | — | + | ND | + | + | — | 61 |
| 7,12-Dimethylbenzanthracene | Sheepshead | — | + | ND | ND | + | — | 61 |
| 1,2,4-Trimethylnaphthalene | Rainbow trout | + | — | ND | ND | ND | ND | 37,104 |
| | Rainbow trout | — | — | ND | ND | ND | ND | 45 |
| Phenanthrene | Rainbow trout | — | — | ND | ND | ND | ND | 87 |
| | Cunner[e] | ND | — | ND | ND | ND | ND | 87 |
| Pyrene | Rainbow trout | + | + | ND | ND | ND | ND | 45 |
| | Cunner[e] | ND | ND | ND | ND | ND | ND | 87 |
| Fluoranthrene | Rainbow trout | — | — | ND | ND | ND | ND | 45 |
| Pyrene and fluoranthrene | Rainbow trout[e] | + | — | ND | ND | ND | ND | 45 |
| Chrysene | Rainbow trout | + | — | ND | ND | ND | ND | 45 |
| Benzo(a)pyrene | Rainbow trout | + | + | ND | ND | ND | ND | 45 |
| | Rainbow trout[e] | + | + | ND | ND | ND | ND | 45 |
| Dibenzothiophene | Cunner[e] | ND | — | ND | ND | ND | ND | 87 |

[a] AH = Aniline hydroxylase activity.
[b] — = No effect or decrease.
[c] + = Increase.
[d] ND — Not determined or reported.
[e] Water exposure; all others i.p. or p.o.

solubilized hepatic microsomes from these animals contained two cytochrome(s) P-450 fractions, one of which had an absorption maximum of 448 nm. As alluded to earlier, it was postulated that this lower proportion of cytochrome P-448 in a dominant environment of cytochrome P-450 may account for the lack of a blue shift toward 448 nm in the induced microsomes. Furthermore, these investigators demonstrated differential *in vitro* effects of αNF on AHH activity in polycyclic aromatic hydrocarbon-induced and control sheepshead and skate, suggesting that the induction produced in fish was similar to that observed in mammalian hepatic microsomes after treatment with 3-MC. While the nature of the control (constitutive) cytochrome(s) P-450 may vary among species of fish studied, there appears to be no question that polycyclic aromatic hydrocarbons induce a spectrum of MO activities that are similar to those induced by this class of inducer in mammals. Whether or not there are discrete differences between specific polycyclic aromatic hydrocarbon inducers in fish is a question that has not yet been addressed.

While treatment of the experimental animals in the above studies has been predominantly by the i.p. route, an important toxicological consideration concerns whether or not hepatic MO enzymes in fish can be induced by exposure to the chemicals under study via the diet or in the water. While experiments in which administration of inducers by the i.p. route have been valuable and have made important contributions to the characterization of the induction response, only recently has it been demonstrated that fish can be induced by water exposure to polycyclic aromatic hydrocarbons (45). An important consideration in experiments involving water exposure to inducers is the bioaccumulation factor of the inducer in organs in which MO induction is to be studied. Thus, if it is accepted that a given compound must be present in the liver at a certain minimum concentration for a specified time period in order to result in induction, the bioaccumulation factor of that particular inducer in the organ under study is an important determinant of the threshold levels in water that are necessary to affect induction.

## Crude Oil and its Components

There have been several suggestions in the recent literature that AHH activity in fish liver may provide a useful tool in assessing previous exposure to water contamination by petroleum-derived polycyclic aromatic hydrocarbons (71,86,88,107,124). Although the interpretation of data from this type of study is problematic, due to inherent variations in MO activities among wild populations, as well as the possibility of detecting polycyclic aromatic hydrocarbon-type induction produced by other compounds (halogenated hydrocarbons), several studies have demonstrated elevated AHH activities in hepatic tissues from fish sampled from "contaminated waters." It should be noted that pike (*Esox lucius*) from heavily polluted waters have been shown to possess only 20% of the hepatic microsomal AHH activity of control animals, and this has been ascribed to the presence of hepatotoxins in this environment (5). Thus, whether or not monitoring of MO activity in aquatic species can be used as a reliable measure of petroleum contamination is still open to question.

In the laboratory, it has been possible to demonstrate elevated AHH activity in liver microsomes from rainbow trout exposed to benzo(a)pyrene in water and from the cunner exposed to slicks of Venezuelan TiaJuana crude oil (45,123). While the specific components of the crude oil that are responsible for AHH induction have not been identified, there appear to be several chromatographic fractions capable of inducing MO enzymes when injected into rainbow trout intraperitoneally. Several crude oil components have been studied for their ability to produce MO induction when exposed to fish via the water route (45). Many of these compounds, including benzene, xylene, naphthalene, phenanthrene, pyrene, and fluoranthrene, did not significantly elevate levels of AHH activity in livers of cunner or rainbow trout. These experiments are difficult to interpret because some of these compounds are poor inducers in mammals, and complete dose-response curves were not constructed, either by water exposure or by the i.p. route. Some confusion in the literature exists concerning whether certain polycyclic aromatic hydrocarbons are inducers of MO in fish, and this problem has arisen because experimental protocols have been designed with different questions in mind. For the investigator interested in the characterization of induction processes in fish, it is important to determine if induction occurs at any dose given, regardless of the route of administration; on the other hand, for environmental considerations, it is important to know whether induction occurs in a given species exposed to polycyclic aromatic hydrocarbons in the diet or at certain water concentrations. It should, therefore, be kept in mind that mechanistic studies are concerned primarily with molecular structure and intrinsic biological activity of chemicals, while environmental studies are more appropriately directed toward parameters related to dose-effect relationships, such as bioaccumulation factors, water, and food chain levels of chemicals that may reflect environmental exposure conditions. Experiments should be designed to determine if a compound is an inducer through appropriate dose ranging studies; after the intrinsic activity is established, the relevance of these observations to environmental exposure conditions must be a primary objective.

## HALOGENATED ORGANIC CHEMICALS

### Biphenyls

The polyhalogenated biphenyls are wide-spread environmental contaminants known to accumulate in aquatic species (68,70). Extensive studies in mammals have suggested that crude polyhalogenated biphenyl mixtures, for example Aroclors and FireMaster BP6, are capable of inducing both cytochrome(s) P-450 and P-448-linked MO activities (8,14,31,33,75). Further studies have indicated that the type of induction observed is dependent on the halogen substitution pattern of the biphenyls (47,94). Simplistically, congeners substituted in the 2-,6-,2'-, or 6'-position are noncoplanar and induce cytochrome(s) P-450, while congeners unsubstituted in these positions are coplanar and induce cytochrome(s) P-448. Several workers have investigated the effects of polyhalogenated biphenyl mixtures on aquatic species, but few attempts have been made to identify which congeners are able to induce MO activity in fish.

It has been demonstrated that *p*-nitroanisole-o-demethylation and hemoprotein(s) P-450 content in hepatic microsomes of rainbow trout increase after administration of the PCB mixture Clophen A-50 (73). Similar studies in the channel catfish revealed increases in cytochrome(s) P-450, b5, and NADPH cytochrome c reductase activity after administration of Aroclor 1254, but no increases in aminopyrine-N-demethylation were observed in this study (74). Further work with the channel catfish indicated that significant increases in hepatic MO activity could be observed using higher doses of Aroclor 1254; and in this study, aminopyrine-N-demethylase activity appeared to be stimulated threefold (69). Other investigators have also demonstrated a slight induction of aminopyrine-N-demethylation (1.7-fold) and aniline hydroxylation (1.4-fold) in the channel catfish after administration of Aroclor 1254 (59).

AHH activity was stimulated in the liver of coho salmon (*Oncorhynchus kisutch*) by Aroclor 1242 at 1 ppm in the diet for 60 days (49). Induction of ECOD has been demonstrated in brook trout (*Salvelinus fontinalis*) after Aroclor 1254 pretreatment, but with the dosing regimen used, no increase in cytochrome(s) P-450 content or in aniline hydroxylation was observed (3).

Recent work has indicated that both Aroclors 1254 and 1242 are potent inducers of AHH, ECOD, and EROD in the rainbow trout. Neither mixture, however, was found to affect the N-demethylation of ethylmorphine (a phenobarbital-type substrate). After a single injection of 150 mg/kg of Aroclor 1254, MO activity remained elevated for at least 21 days, and SDS-PAGE of hepatic microsomes obtained from rainbow trout pretreated with Aroclor 1242 exhibited an intense Coomassie blue-staining band at 57,000 daltons. This also was seen after pretreatment of rainbow trout with βNF (38).

These studies appear to indicate that the so-called "mixed" induction properties of the PCBs seen in mammals were not fully expressed in fish, and hence the inducing potential of several pure

PCB congeners has been studied. Table 4 illustrates the results obtained from rainbow trout using these pure congeners.

The crude PCB mixtures Aroclor 1254 and 1242 induced ECOD and EROD, but not BeND. In the rat, all three of these reactions were induced by the PCB mixtures. The coplanar PCBs (3,4,3',4'-tetra- and 3,4,5,3',4'-pentachlorobiphenyl) were good inducers of ECOD and EROD; however, the noncoplanar isomers (2,4,2',4'-tetra-, and 2,4,5,2',4',5'-hexachlorobiphenyl) were without effect (Table 4). None of the congeners examined altered BeND significantly, and these results were similar to those obtained with polybrominated biphenyl (PBB) congeners. SDS-PAGE of hepatic microsomes of rainbow trout revealed an induced protein band(s) with a molecular weight of 57,000 daltons after pretreatment with Aroclor 1254, Aroclor 1242, or 3,4,3',4'-tetrachlorobiphenyl (Fig. 3). There were no changes in the electrophoretic microsomal protein profiles after treatment of rainbow trout with the noncoplanar con-

TABLE 4. *Induction of hepatic microsomal MO activity in the rainbow trout by various PCB congeners*

| Treatment[a] | BeND[b] | ECOD[c] nmole/min/mg protein | EROD[c] |
|---|---|---|---|
| Corn oil | 1.05 | $0.023 \pm .003$ | $0.025 \pm .009$ |
| | 1.23 | | |
| Aroclor 1254 | 0.51 | — | $0.365 \pm .100$[e] |
| Aroclor 1242 | 1.40 | $0.186 \pm .053$[e] | $0.608 \pm .379$[e] |
| 2,4,2',4'-tetra | 1.08 | $0.045 \pm .008$ | $0.085 \pm .057$ |
| 3,4,3',4'-tetra | 1.37 | $0.148 \pm .015$[e] | $0.519 \pm .101$[e] |
| 3,4,5,3',4'-penta | 0.47 | $0.647 \pm .078$[e] | $0.356 \pm .051$[e] |
| 2,4,5,2',4',5'-hexa | N.D.[d] | $0.030 \pm .001$ | $0.010 \pm .007$ |

[a]Animals were pretreated i.p. with a single injection of each agent at a dose of 150 mg/kg, and sacrificed 5 days thereafter.
[b]Values obtained using pooled microsomes from 5 fish.
[c]Values represent mean $\pm$ SE, $n = 8$.
[d]Not detectable.
[e]Significantly different from corn oil-pretreated controls, $p < 0.05$.
Some of the data in Table 4 are from Elcombe et al., ref. 36.

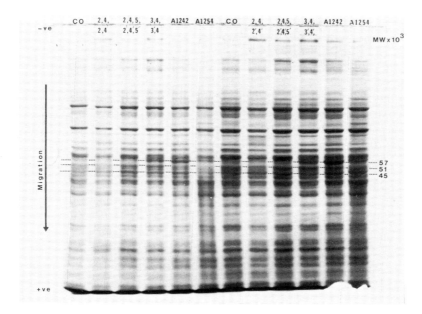

**FIG. 3.** SDS-PAGE of hepatic microsomes from rainbow trout pretreated with various PCB congeners. The first six columns represent loadings of 45 μg protein; the last six, 90 μg protein. The horizontal lines indicate MWs of 57,000, 51,000, and 45,000 daltons. CO: Corn oil-treated controls.

geners 2,4,2′,4′-tetra-, or 2,4,5,2′,4′,5′-hexachlorobiphenyl. These studies support the hypothesis expressed earlier that phenobarbital-type induction does not appear to occur in the rainbow trout.

Other studies have indicated that 4-chlorobiphenyl and 2,5,2′,5′-tetrachlorobiphenyl were not effective in inducing cytochrome(s) P-450 or paranitroanisole-o-demethylation in the rainbow trout (42). However, these investigators did demonstrate increases in both cytochrome(s) P-450 content and paranitroanisole demethylation by 2,4,5,2′,4′,5′-hexachlorobiphenyl. Similar results have been reported for 2,4,5,2′,5′-pentachlorobiphenyl in coho salmon (48). The ability of these noncoplanar PCB congeners to induce in fish is in conflict with many studies showing the refractivity of these animals to phenobarbital-type induction. Many "pure" PCB congeners are contaminated with potent inducers, such as TCDF, and conflicting results of induction profiles in the rat have been explained on the basis of impure inducing agents (46).

FireMaster BP6, a commercial mixture of PBBs, is a potent inducer of MO activity in mammals (32), and studies suggest that a broad spectrum of MO activities are stimulated in a similar manner to that seen after PCB treatment. In the rainbow trout, FireMaster BP6 induced hepatic ECOD, EROD, and AHH, but not ethylmorphine-N-demethylation (37).

Recent work using rainbow trout and pure PBB congeners have indicated similar patterns of induction to those seen with the PCBs. Table 5 illustrates such data. Only FireMaster BP6 and the coplanar congeners elevated ECOD and EROD significantly; BeND was unaffected by all compounds studied. Interestingly, the pure 2,4,5,3',4',5'-hexabromobiphenyl has been shown to induce both cytochrome(s) P-450 and P-448 in the rat, suggesting it to be a true "mixed" inducer (30). However, only slight and insignificant cytochrome(s) $P_1$-450-type induction was observed, in studies in the

TABLE 5. *Induction of hepatic microsomal MO activity in the rainbow trout by various PBB congeners*

| Treatment[a] | BeND[b] | ECOD[c] nmole/min/mg protein | EROD[c] |
|---|---|---|---|
| Corn oil | 1.36 | 0.050 ± .007 | 0.029 ± .006 |
| FireMaster BP6 | 1.50 | 0.126 ± .043 | 0.391 ± .182[e] |
| 2,4,5,2',4',5'-hexa | 1.42 | 0.019 ± .007 | 0.019 ± .008 |
| 2,4,5,3',4',5'-hexa | 1.31 | 0.096 ± .011 | 0.052 ± .013 |
| 3,4,5,3',4',5'-hexa | ND[d] | 0.121 ± .051[e] | 0.182 ± .102[e] |
| 2,3,4,5,2',4',5'-hepta | 1.80 | 0.041 ± .007 | 0.017 ± .002 |

[a]Animals were pretreated i.p. with a single injection of each agent at a dose of 150 mg/kg, and sacrificed 5 days thereafter.
[b]Values obtained using pooled microsomes from 5 fish.
[c]Values represent mean ± SE, $n = 8$.
[d]Not determined.
[e]Significantly different from corn oil-pretreated controls, $p < 0.05$.

rainbow trout with this congener, and there was no discernable effect on BeND activity.

## Dioxins

Dioxins are produced by side reactions in the manufacture of chemicals, such as 2,4,5-trichlorophenoxyacetic acid, and, as such, are found as contaminants in many commercial preparations (84). Some of the chlorinated dioxins are highly toxic and are also potent inducers of cytochrome P-448-mediated MO activity in mammals (47). Few studies have addressed the effects of these chemicals in fish, but induction of hepatic AHH in several marine fish has been reported after TCDD treatment (93).

Several recent investigations have shown TCDD to be a potent inducer of cytochrome $P_1$-450-type activities in the rainbow trout (Table 6). Following a single injection of TCDD (2 μg/kg), an increase in ECOD and EROD was seen, and these elevated activities were maintained for at least 3 weeks. TCDD was also found to increase total hepatic hemoprotein(s) P-450 content, but BeND was unaffected by TCDD pretreatment (122).

TABLE 6. *Effects of TCDD on hepatic microsomal MO activity in the rainbow trout*

| Treatment | Days after treatment | EROD[a] | ECOD[a] |
|---|---|---|---|
| | | (nmole/min/mg protein) | |
| Corn oil | 3 | 0.014 ± 0.014 | 0.025 ± 0.013 |
| TCDD (2 μg/kg) | 3 | 0.966 ± 0.841[b] | 0.103 ± 0.076[b] |
| Corn oil | 6 | 0.013 ± 0.001 | 0.031 ± 0.009 |
| TCDD | 6 | 1.561 ± 0.650 | 0.272 ± 0.169[b] |
| Corn oil | 13 | 0.009 ± 0.004 | 0.036 ± 0.058 |
| TCDD | 13 | 1.23 ± 0.4[b] | 0.467 ± 0.089[b] |
| Corn oil | 21 | 0.015 ± 0.007 | 0.003 ± 0.002 |
| TCDD | 21 | 5.910 ± 1.35[b] | 0.139 ± 0.096[b] |

[a]Values represent mean ± SD, $n = 6$.
[b]Significantly different from corn oil-pretreated controls, $p < 0.05$.

SDS-PAGE of microsomes obtained from the livers of TCDD-treated fish revealed an enhanced 57,000 dalton band, and its intensity correlated with the degree of induction of ECOD and EROD.

## Mirex, Kepone, and DDT

Kepone and Mirex have been suggested to induce cytochrome(s) P-450 profiles in mammals different from those observed with either phenobarbital or 3-MC. Specifically, Kepone administration to rodents has been demonstrated to enhance cytochrome(s) P-450 content and stimulate hepatic microsomal MO activities similar to phenobarbital (40,65,80,81). However, Kepone also resulted in an increase in both type I and type II ligand binding to cytochrome(s) P-450, a shift in the Soret $\lambda$maximum of carboxyferrohemoprotein(s) complex from 450 to 449 nm, and a different warfarin metabolite profile from that observed following phenobarbital administration (40,65).

Mirex treatment of rats resulted in induction of microsomal BeND and ethylmorphine-N-demethylase activities as seen with the barbiturate inducers (79,113), but also resembled 3-MC with respect to a slight shift in the cytochrome(s) P-450 $\lambda$max and the *in vitro* microsomal metabolism of warfarin (65). However, neither Kepone nor Mirex enhanced the activity of microsomal biphenyl-2-hydroxylation relative to biphenyl-4-hydroxylation as observed with many 3-MC-type inducers.

At the doses administered to rainbow trout, neither Kepone (5 mg/kg) nor Mirex (25 and 40 mg/kg) stimulated hepatic microsomal BeND, ECOD, EROD, or NADPH cytochrome c reductase activities or cytochrome(s) P-450 content (122). This is unlikely to be due to a problem of bioavailability since gas chromatographic analysis indicated the presence of these agents in liver extracts of pretreated fish. Furthermore, at a dose of 10 mg/kg to channel catfish, Kepone did not potentiate $CCl_4$ hepatotoxicity as has been demonstrated in the rat (28,29), although the relationship between potentiation of hepatotoxicity and MO induction has not been elucidated.

While both Kepone and Mirex have been demonstrated to possess some inducing properties similar to those observed with 3-MC in mammals, no effect on cytochrome(s) $P_1$-450-type activities or SDS-PAGE was apparent in fish, suggesting these agents to resemble phenobarbital-type inducers in these animals.

The insecticide DDT and its metabolite DDE have been demonstrated to be potent, long-acting inducers of the hepatic microsomal MO system in mammals (118). Coadministration of DDT with phenobarbital or 3-MC generally resulted in additive effects on *in vitro* MO activity (117), but the substrates chosen for study were not specific indicators of cytochrome(s) P-450 or $P_1$-450 induction, and later studies suggested DDT to resemble the barbiturate-type inducing agents (118).

The oral administration of DDT to rainbow trout (2.5 mg/kg on alternate days for 36 days) resulted in a slight but significant induction of aminopyrine-N-demethylation but had no effect on the *p*-hydroxylation of aniline (35). However, early studies (16) suggested DDT to be ineffective as an inducer of MO activity in fish, and more recent work (2) has demonstrated a lack of effect of DDT or DDE on cytochrome(s) P-450 content, aniline hydroxylase, ECOD, and aldrin epoxidase activities in brook trout following the oral administration of 10 doses of DDT (1.5 mg) or 12 doses of DDE (1.7 mg). It therefore appears that the MO system of fish is relatively insensitive to induction by DDT-type agents when compared to the response to these chemicals in other species. Furthermore, whether the induction of aminopyrine-N-demethylation by DDT in early experiments (35) may have been the result of contamination of the chemical must also be considered.

## CONSEQUENCES OF INDUCTION

### Induction in Nature

A question germane to aquatic toxicology in environmental interests is whether or not induction occurs among wild fish populations and its significance. Although induction of MO activity by xenobiotic chemicals in nature implies either water or dietary uptake of the inducer, very few experiments have been designed to study induction under simulated natural conditions. There are reports, however, that indicate that certain species of fish have elevated hepatic AHH activity when exposed to crude oil or certain petroleum fractions under laboratory conditions. The results of such studies confirm and strengthen the hypothesis that the state or level of certain MO enzymes in the livers from wild fish may be a relative indicator of their exposure to inducers in the aquatic environment, and it has been suggested that levels of MO activity in fish be used as a biological monitor for exposure to polycyclic aromatic hydrocarbons. However, from the little that is known about the actions of inducers in fish, it is obvious that levels of AHH activity in liver would not be a specific indicator of polycyclic aromatic hydrocarbon exposure, since AHH activity can also be elevated by other inducers of the 3-MC class, including certain PCB and PBB isomers and TCDD. From the physiological and ecological points of view, the consequences of MO induction have yet to be explored, and questions related to the effect of MO induction on biotransformation pathways, acute and chronic toxicity of chemicals, and on steroid metabolism have only recently been addressed.

## Biotransformation Pathways for Xenobiotic Chemicals

With few exceptions, most of the studies described in the previous sections have dealt with the effect of various classes of inducers on the levels of activity of a variety of MO enzymes. The protocols involved in most of these experiments have been quite similar, involving pretreatment of the species in question with various inducers, with subsequent measurement of the rates of a variety of MO-catalyzed reactions in either microsomes or other liver fractions *in vitro*. It is known, however, from the mammalian literature that the qualitative as well as quantitative aspects of MO-catalyzed biotransformation pathways can be altered, depending on whether the inducer is phenobarbital- or 3-MC-like. Thus, it is well established that various hepatic MO inducers have the ability to produce significant changes in the metabolite patterns produced upon incubation of biphenyl and benzo(a)pyrene with hepatic microsomes prepared from pretreated animals (27,95). This induced positional selectivity of monooxygenation appears to be specific for certain classes of inducers, and, in recent years, has taken on additional significance since it was demonstrated that certain metabolic pathways can lead to the formation of biologically active metabolites that are more toxic than the parent compound. *In vitro* benzo(a)pyrene metabolite patterns have been intensively studied in some cases to characterize and classify other chemicals that are inducers. Benzo(a)pyrene metabolite patterns have been studied by high pressure liquid chromatography in microsomes from only a few species of fish. Microsomes prepared from control lake trout (*Salmo trutta*) produced a metabolite pattern that was dominated by a 9,10-dihydrodiol, 7,8-dihydrodiol, and 3-phenol, and this pattern was more closely related to that seen in liver microsomes prepared from 3-MC-treated rats as compared to control rats (7). Although inducers were not used in this study with lake trout, the similarities in the benzo(a)pyrene metabolite patterns between control trout microsomes and microsomes from 3-MC-treated rat liver strongly suggest that the trout liver constitutive (control) cytochrome(s) P-450 are closely related catalytically to polycyclic aromatic hydrocarbon-induced cytochrome(s) $P_1$-450 of rat liver (7). Treatment of the little skate with 1,2,3,4-dibenzanthracene resulted in a 10- to 15-fold increase in the rate of production of benzo(a)pyrene metabolites using hepatic microsomes *in vitro*, and the metabolite pattern observed with the induced microsomes was qualitatively similar to that seen using control microsomes (12). The only significant difference between the control and induced benzo(a)pyrene metabolite patterns in the little skate was in the quinone plus epoxide region; this was attributed to the accumulation of benzo(a)pyrene 4,5,-oxide in the incubation mixtures. Pretreatment of channel catfish with 3-MC produced significant changes in the *in vitro* metabolism of benzo(a)pyrene by isolated hepatic microsomes. Although only a modest increase in overall metabolism was observed, large and significant increases in the production of 9,10-diol, 7,8-diol, and quinones were observed in the induced microsomes (60).

Few studies are available concerning the effect of induction on the metabolism and disposition of xenobiotic chemicals in fish *in vivo*, although it has been reported that the biliary excretion of [14]C-2-methylnaphthalene metabolites was increased approximately three-fold by pretreatment of rainbow trout with 2,3,-benzanthracene (104). A similar effect has been noted in rainbow trout exposed to 1,2,4-trichlorobenzene and 2-methylnaphthalene after induction with βNF (83). In addition to an increased biliary excretion of these compounds, analysis by thin layer chromatography indicated that there may have been changes in the pattern of biliary metabolites due to hepatic enzyme induction (83).

## Toxicity of Chemicals

It is well known from studies in mammals that induction of the hepatic MO system can alter the toxicity of certain chemicals resulting in an increase or a decrease in toxicity, depending on the chemical and the biotransformation reaction. Qualitative differences in metabolic pathways for certain compounds leading to increased toxicity have been observed after induction; in some cases, this has been attributed to induction of cytochrome(s) P-450-linked MOs that lead to the increased formation of reactive metabolites, such as benzo(a)pyrene-7,8-dihydrodiol-9,10-epoxide and aflatoxin $B_1$-2,3-oxide. On the other hand, increases in metabolism as a consequence of induction can result in a more rapid conversion to a less toxic species, and this, along with enhanced excretion, can reduce the toxicity of a given compound.

While the effects of MO induction on toxicity have been less well studied in fish than in mammals, it has been demonstrated that covalent binding of metabolites to DNA occurs after incubation of benzo(a)pyrene with microsomes prepared from coho salmon and lake trout liver (7,120) and that induction with 3-MC increases covalent binding by 10- to 50-fold (120). While this metabolic activation and covalent binding have not been demonstrated to be a toxic effect per se in fish, by analogy with studies in mammals, the implication is that binding to DNA may be directly related to mutagenicity and carcinogenicity.

Aflatoxin $B_1$ (AFB$_1$) has shown to be a potent hepatocarcinogen in rainbow trout (99), and it is thought that this compound is metabolized to an ultimate carcinogen by the hepatic MO system in rat liver (114). Although the precise mechanism is unknown, dietary treatment of rainbow trout with the PCB mixture, Aroclor 1254, significantly reduced the incidence of liver tumors due to AFB$_1$ (58). There are several possible explanations for this observation, one of which proposes the induction of hepatic MO leading to metabolism of AFB$_1$ to a less carcinogenic compound (58).

## Hormone Metabolism

Numerous studies in mammals have demonstrated significant correlations between various physiological conditions and hepatic microsomal cytochrome(s) P-450 content and associated enzymic activities. Since the metabolism of both xenobiotic chemicals and steroid hormones appears to be mediated via the cytochrome(s) P-450-dependent MO system, alterations in this system may affect sex steroid metabolism and, thus, reproductive function as well.

A number of studies in mammals and birds have suggested this to be the case in that exposure to environmental contaminants known to induce hepatic microsomal MO activities alter sex hormone metabolism, and, in turn, reproductive processes (26,34,91,96). Elevated sex steroid levels are also necessary to maintain vitellogenesis and spermatogenesis in fish, and since an active cytochrome(s) P-450 MO system has been demonstrated in these animals, it is possible that an alteration in this system may affect reproductive function. PCBs, potent inducers of MO activity in the rainbow trout, have been shown to cause a reduction in plasma levels of the sex steroids (100) and a stimulation of the *in vitro* 11β-hydroxylation of testosterone by testicular tissue in these animals (43). Furthermore, it has been demonstrated that the administration of 3-MC or Clophen A50 to rainbow trout altered the hepatic microsomal cytochrome(s) P-450-mediated metabolism of 4-androstene-3,17-dione *in vitro* (55). The administration of phenobarbital to these animals had no effect on androstenedione metabolism, further supporting the observation that fish are refractive to induction by cytochrome(s) P-450-type inducers. Whether administration of various environmental contaminants alters plasma steroid profiles and gonadal condition, however, has not been investigated.

Since the metabolism of steroid hormones may be modified by inducers of hepatic microsomal MO activity and since various investigators have demonstrated that fish from contaminated environments have elevated MO activities when compared to their counterparts from pristine waters, the effects of water-borne chemicals known to be inducers of the MO system on reproductive processes in fish may be of environmental and toxicological significance.

## ACKNOWLEDGMENTS

Supported in part by grants from the U.S. Environmental Protection Agency, The University of Wisconsin Sea Grant Institute, and the National Institute of Environmental Health Sciences (ES 01080 and the Aquatic Biomedical Research Center Grant ES 01985).

## REFERENCES

1. Adamson, R. H. (1967): Drug metabolism in marine vertebrates. *Fed. Proc.*, 26:1,047–1,055.
2. Addison, R. F., Zinck, M. E., and Willis, D. E. (1977): Mixed-function oxidase in trout liver: Absence of induction following feed of p,p'-DDT or p,p'-DDE. *Comp. Biochem. Pharmacol.*, 75C:39–43.
3. Addison, R. F., Zinck, M. E., and Willis, D. E. (1978): Induction of hepatic mixed-function oxidase (MFO) enzymes in trout (*Salvelinus fontinalis*) by feeding Aroclor 1254 or 3-methylcholanthrene. *Comp. Biochem. Physiol.*, 61:323–325.
4. Ahokas, J. T. (1979): Cytochrome P-450 in fish liver microsomes and carcinogen activation. In: *Pesticide and Xenobiotic Metabolism in Aquatic Organisms*, edited by M. A. Q. Khan, J. J. Lech, and J. J. Menn, pp. 279–296. American Chemical Society, Washington, D. C.
5. Ahokas, J. T., Karki, N. T., Oikari, A., and Soivio, A. (1976): Mixed function monooxygenase of fish as an indicator of pollution of aquatic environment by industrial effluent. *Bull. Environ. Contam. Toxicol.*, 16:270–274.

6. Ahokas, J. T., Pelkonen, O., and Karki, N. T. (1977): Characterization of benzo(a)pyrene hydroxylase of trout liver. *Cancer Res.*, 37:3,737–3,743.
7. Ahokas, J. T., Saarni, H., Nebert, D. W., and Pelkonen, O. (1979): The *in vitro* metabolism and covalent binding of benzo(a)pyrene to DNA catalyzed by trout liver microsomes. *Chem. Biol. Interact.*, 25:103–111.
8. Alvares, A. P., Bickers, D. R., and Kappas, A. (1973): Polychlorinated biphenyls: A new type of inducer of cytochrome P-448 in the liver. *Proc. Natl. Acad. Sci., U.S.*, 70:1,321–1,325.
9. Alvares, A. P., Schilling, G., Levin, W., and Kuntzman, R. (1967): Studies on the induction of CO-binding pigments in liver microsomes by phenobarbital and 3-methylcholanthrene. *Biochem. Biophys. Res. Commun.*, 29:521–526.
10. Alvares, A. P., and Siekevitz, P. (1973): Gel electrophoresis of partially purified cytochrome P-450 from liver microsomes of various treated rats. *Biochem. Biophys. Res. Commun.*, 54:923–929.
11. Balk, L., Meijer, J., Siedegard, J., Morganstein, R., and Depierre, J. W. (1980): Initial characterization of drug-metabolizing systems in the liver of the northern pike, *Esox lucius*. *Drug Metab. Dispos.*, 8:98–103.
12. Bend, J. R., Ball, L. M., Elmamlouk, T. H., James, M. O., and Philpot, R. M. (1979): Microsomal mixed-function oxidation in untreated and polycyclic aromatic hydrocarbon-treated marine fish. In: *Pesticide and Xenobiotic Metabolism in Aquatic Organisms*, edited by M. A. Q. Khan, J. J. Lech, and J. J. Menn, pp. 279–318. American Chemical Society, Washington D. C.
13. Bend, J. R., and James, M. O. (1979): Xenobiotic metabolism in marine and freshwater species. *Biochem. Biophys. Perspect. Mar. Biol.*, 4:125–188.
14. Bickers, D. R., Harber, L. C., Kappas, A., and Alvares, A. P. (1972): Polychlorinated biphenyls: Comparative effects of high and low chlorine containing Aroclors on hepatic mixed-function oxidase. *Res. Commun. Chem. Pathol. Pharmacol.*, 3:505–512.
15. Birnbaum, L. S., Baird, M. B., and Massie, H. R. (1976): Pregnenolone-16α-carbonitrile-inducible cytochrome P-450 in rat liver. *Res. Commun. Chem. Pathol. Pharmacol.*, 15:553–562.
16. Buhler, D. R., and Rasmusson, M. E. (1968): The oxidation of drugs by fishes. *Comp. Biochem. Physiol.*, 25:223–239.
17. Burke, M. D., and Mayer, R. T. (1974): Ethoxyresorufin: Direct fluorometric assay of a microsomal o-dealkylation which is preferentially inducible by 3-methylcholanthrene. *Drug. Metab. Dispos.*, 2:583–588.
18. Burns, K. (1976): Microsomal mixed-function oxidases in an estuarine fish, *Fundulus heteroclitus*, and their induction as a result of environmental contamination. *Comp. Biochem. Physiol.*, 53B:443–446.
19. Chambers, J. E., and Yarbrough, J. D. (1976): Xenobiotic biotransformation systems in fishes. *Comp. Biochem. Physiol.*, 55C:77–84.
20. Chambers, J. E., and Yarbrough, J. D. (1979): A seasonal study of microsomal mixed-function oxidase components in insecticide-resistant and susceptible mosquitofish, *Gambusia affinis*. *Toxicol. Appl. Pharmacol.*, 48:497–507.

21. Chan, T. M., Gillett, J. W., and Terriere, L. C. (1967): Interaction between microsomal electron transport systems of trout and male rat in cyclodiene epoxidation. *Comp. Biochem. Physiol.*, 20:731–742.

22. Chevion, M., Stegeman, J. J., Piesach, J., and Blumberg, W. E. (1977): Electron paramagnetic resonance studies on hepatic microsomal cytochrome P-450 from a marine teleost fish. *Life Sci.*, 20:895–900.

23. Conney, A. H. (1967): Pharmacological implications of microsomal enzyme induction. *Pharmacol. Rev.*, 19:317–364.

24. Conney, A. H., Davison, C., Gastel, R., and Burns, J. J. (1960): Adaptive increases in drug-metabolizing enzymes induced by phenobarbital and other drugs. *J. Pharmacol. Exp. Ther.*, 130:1–8.

25. Conney, A. H., and Gilmann, A. G. (1963): Puromycin inhibition of enzyme induction by 3-methylcholanthrene and phenobarbital. *J. Biol. Chem.*, 238:3,682–3,685.

26. Conney, A. H., Levin, W., Jacobson, M., and Kuntzman, R. (1973): Effects of drugs and environmental chemicals on steroid metabolism. *Clin. Pharmacol. Ther.*, 14:727–741.

27. Creaven, P. J., and Parke, D. V. (1966): The stimulation of hydroxylation by carcinogenic and noncarcinogenic compounds. *Biochem. Pharmacol.*, 15:7–13.

28. Curtis, L. R., and Mehendale, H. M. (1980): Refractoriness of channel catfish to Kepone potentiated $CCl_4$ hepatotoxicity. *Toxicol. Appl. Pharmacol. (Abstract)*53:A79.

29. Curtis, L. R., Williams, W. L., and Mehendale, H. M. (1979): Potentiation of the hepatotoxicity of carbon tetrachloride following preexposure to chlordecone (Kepone) in the male rat. *Toxicol. Appl. Pharmacol.*, 51:283–293.

30. Dannon, G. A., Moore, R. W., Besaw, L. C., and Aust, S. D. (1978): 2,4,5,3',4',5'-hexabromobiphenyl is both a 3-MC- and PB-type inducer of microsomal drug metabolizing enzymes. *Biochem. Biophys. Res. Commun.*, 85:450–458.

31. Dent, J. G. (1977): Stimulation of hepatic microsomal metabolism in mice by a mixture of polybrominated biphenyls. *J. Toxicol. Environ. Health*, 6:651–661.

32. Dent, J. G. (1978): Characteristics of cytochrome P-450 and mixed-function oxidase enzymes following treatment with PBBs. *Environ. Health Perspect.*, 23: 301–308.

33. Dent, J. G., Netter, K. J., and Gibson, J. E. (1976): The induction of hepatic microsomal metabolism in rats following acute administration of a mixture of polybrominated biphenyls. *Toxicol. Appl. Pharmacol.*, 38:237–249.

34. Derr, S. K. (1978): *In vivo* metabolism of exogenous progesterones by PCB-treated female rats. *Bull. Environ. Contam. Toxicol.*, 19:729–732.

35. DeWaide, J. H. (1971): *Metabolism of Xenobiotics*. Ph.D. Thesis, University of Nijmegen, The Netherlands.

36. Elcombe, C. R., Franklin, R. B., and Lech, J. J. (1979): Induction of hepatic microsomal enzymes in rainbow trout. In: *Pesticide and Xenobiotic Metab-*

*olism in Aquatic Organisms*, edited by M. A. Q. Khan, J. J. Lech, and J. J. Menn, pp. 319–337. American Chemical Society, Washington, D.C.

37. Elcombe, C. R., and Lech, J. J. (1978): Induction of monooxygenation in rainbow trout by polybrominated biphenyls: A comparative study. *Environ. Health Perspect.*, 23:309–314.

38. Elcombe, C. R., and Lech, J. J. (1979): Induction and characterization of hemoprotein(s) P-450 and monooxygenation in rainbow trout (*Salmo gairdneri*). *Toxicol. Appl. Pharmacol.*, 49:437–450.

39. Elshourbagy, N. A., and Guzelian, P. S. (1980): Separation, purification, and characterization of a novel form of hepatic cytochrome P-450 from rats treated with pregnenolone-16α-carbonitrile. *J. Biol. Chem.*, 255:1,279–1,285.

40. Fabacher, D. L., and Hodgson, E. (1976): Induction of hepatic mixed-function oxidase enzymes in adult and neonatal mice by Kepone and Mirex. *Toxicol. Appl. Pharmacol.*, 38:71–77.

41. Feuer, G. (1979): Action of pregnancy and various progesterones on hepatic microsomal activities. *Drug Metab. Rev.*, 9:147–169.

42. Forlin, L., and Lidman, U. (1978): Effects of Clophen A50, 2,5,2',5'-tetra- and 2,4,5,2',4',5'-hexachlorobiphenyl on the mixed-function oxidase system of rainbow trout liver. *Comp. Biochem. Physiol.*, 60C:193–197.

43. Freeman, H. C., and Idler, D. R. (1975): The effect of polychlorinated biphenyl on steroidogenesis and reproduction in the brook trout (*Salvelinus fontinalis*). *Can. J. Biochem.*, 53: 666–670.

44. Gelboin, H. V., and Blackburn, N. R. (1964): The stimulating effect of 3-MC on benzpyrene hydroxylase activity on several rat tissues: Inhibition by Actinomycin D and Puromycin. *Cancer Res.*, 25B:356–359.

45. Gerhart, E. H., and Carlson, R. M. (1978): Hepatic mixed-function oxidase activity in rainbow trout exposed to several polycyclic aromatic compounds. *Environ. Res.*, 17:284–295.

46. Goldstein, J. A., Hass, J. R., Linko, P., and Harvan, D. J. (1978): 2,3,7,8,-tetrachlorodibenzofuran in a commercially available 99% pure polychlorinated biphenyl isomer identified as the inducer of cytochrome P-448 and aryl hydrocarbon hydroxylase in the rat. *Drug Metab. Dispos.*, 6:258–264.

47. Goldstein, J. A., Hickman, P., Bergman, H., McKinney, J. D., and Walker, M. P. (1977): Separation of pure polychlorinated biphenyl isomers into two types of inducers on the basis of induction of cytochrome P-450 or P-448. *Chem. Biol. Interact.*, 17:284–295.

48. Gruger, Jr., E. H., Hruby, T., and Karrick, N. L. (1976): Sublethal effects of structurally related tetrachloro-, pentachloro-, and hexachlorobiphenyl on juvenile coho salmon. *J. Environ. Sci. Tech.*, 10:1,033–1,037.

49. Gruger, Jr., E. H., Wekell, M. M., Numoto, P. T., and Craddock, D. R. (1977): Induction of hepatic aryl hydrocarbon hydroxylase in salmon exposed to petroleum dissolved in seawater and to petroleum and polychlorinated biphenyls, separate and together, in food. *Bull. Environ. Contam. Toxicol.*, 17:512–520.

50. Guengerich, F. P. (1977): Separation and purification of multiple forms of microsomal cytochrome P-450. *J. Biol. Chem.*, 252:3,970–3,979.

51. Guenther, T. M., and Mannering, G. J. (1977): Induction of hepatic mono-oxygenase systems of pregnant rats with phenobarbital and 3-methylchol-anthrene. *Biochem. Pharmacol.*, 26:577–584.
52. Gutman, Y., and Kidron, M. (1971): Liver N-demethylating activity—Temperature effect and phenobarbital induction in different species. *Biochem. Pharmacol.*, 20:3,547–3,549.
53. Hansen, L. G., Kapoor, I. P., and Metcalf, R. L. (1972): Biochemistry of selective toxicity and biodegradability: Comparative o-dealkylation by aquatic organisms. *Comp. Gen. Pharmacol.*, 3:339–344.
54. Hansson, T., and Lidman, U. (1978): Effects of cortisol administration on components of the hepatic microsomal mixed-function oxidase system (MFO) of immature rainbow trout. *Acta Pharmacol. Toxicol.*, 43:6–12.
55. Hansson, T., Rafter, J., and Gustafsson, J. A. (1980): Effects of some common inducers on the hepatic microsomal metabolism of androstenedione in rainbow trout with special reference to cytochrome P-450-dependent enzymes. *Biochem. Pharmacol.*, 29:583–587.
56. Haugen, D. A., Coon, M. J., and Nebert, D. W. (1976): Induction of multiple forms of mouse liver cytochrome P-450: Evidence for genetically controlled *de novo* protein synthesis in response to treatment with β-naphthoflavone or phenobarbital. *J. Biol. Chem.*, 251:1,817–1,828.
57. Haugen, D. A., van der Hoeven, J. A., and Coon, M. J. (1975): Purified liver cytochrome P-450. *J. Biol. Chem.*, 250:3,567–3,570.
58. Hendricks, J. D., Putnam, T. P., Bills, D. D., and Sinnhuber, R. O. (1977): Inhibitory effect of a polychlorinated biphenyl (Aroclor 1254) on aflatoxin $B_1$ carcinogenesis in rainbow trout. *J. Natl. Cancer Inst.*, 59:1,545–1,550.
59. Hill, D. W., Hejtmancik, E., and Camp, B. J. (1976): Induction of hepatic microsomal enzymes by Aroclor 1254 in *Ictalurus punctatus* (Channel Catfish). *Bull. Environ. Contam. Toxicol.*, 16:495–502.
60. Hinton, D. E., Klaunig, J. E., Jack, R. M., Kipsky, M. M., and Trump, B. J. (1981): *In vitro* evaluation of the channel catfish (*Ictalurus punctatus*) as a test species in chemical carcinogenesis studies. In: *Aquatic Toxicology and Hazard Assessment*, 4th Conference, ASTM STP 737, edited by D. R. Branson and K. L. Dickson, pp. 226–238. American Society for Testing and Materials, Chicago, Illinois.
61. James, M. O., and Bend, J. R. (1980): Polycyclic aromatic hydrocarbon induction of cytochrome P-450 dependent mixed-function oxidases in marine fish. *Toxicol. Appl. Pharmacol.*, 54:117–133.
62. James, M. O., and Bend, J. R. (1980): Effect of polynuclear aromatic hydrocarbons and polyhalogenated biphenyls on hepatic mixed-function oxidase activity in marine fish. *Proceedings of EPA Symposium on Polynuclear Aromatic Hydrocarbons in the Marine Environment* (*in press*).
63. James, M. O., Khan, M. A. Q., and Bend, J. R. (1979): Hepatic microsomal mixed-function oxidase activities in several marine species common to coastal Florida. *Comp. Biochem. Physiol.*, 62C:155–164.

64. Jori, A., and Pescador, R. (1974): Strain differences in the induction of soluble and microsomal enzymes by phenobarbital and 3-methylcholanthrene. *Chem. Biol. Interact.*, 8:297–302.
65. Kaminsky, L. S., Piper, L. J., McMartin, D. N., and Fasco, M. J. (1978): Induction of hepatic microsomal cytochrome P-450 by Mirex and Kepone. *Toxicol. Appl. Pharmacol.*, 43:327–338.
66. Kato, R., (1974): Sex-related differences in drug metabolism. *Drug Metab. Rev.*, 3:1–32.
67. Kato, R. (1977): Drug metabolism under pathological and abnormal physiological states in animals and man. *Xenobiotica*, 7:25–92.
68. Kay, K. (1977): Polybrominated biphenyls (PBB): Environmental Contamination in Michigan, 1973–1976. *Environ. Res.*, 13:74–93.
69. Klaunig, J. E., Lipsky, M. M., Trump, B. F., and Hinton, D. E. (1979): Biochemical and ultrastructural changes in teleost liver following subacute exposure to PCB. *J. Environ. Pathol. Toxicol.*, 2:953–963.
70. Koeman, J. H., T. Noever DeBrauw, M. C., and DeVos, R. H. (1969): Chlorinated biphenyls in fish, mussels, and birds from the river Rhine and the Netherlands coastal area. *Nature*, 221:1,126–1,128.
71. Kurelec, B., Britvic, S., Rijavec, M., Muller, W. E. G., and Zahn, R. K. (1977): Benzo(a)pyrene monooxygenase induction in marine fish—Molecular response to oil pollution. *Mar. Biol.*, 44:211–216.
72. Lech, J. J., and Bend, J. R. (1980): The relationship between biotransformation and the toxicity and fate of xenobiotic chemicals in fish. *Environ. Health Perspect.*, 34:115–131.
73. Lidman, U., Forlin, L., Molander, O., and Axelson, G. (1976): Induction of the drug metabolizing system in rainbow trout (*Salmo gairdneri*) liver by polychlorinated biphenyls (PCBs). *Acta Pharmacol. Toxicol.*, 39:262–272.
74. Lipsky, M. M., Klaunig, J. E., and Hinton, D. E. (1978): Comparison of acute response to polychlorinated biphenyl in liver of rat and channel catfish: A biochemical and morphological study. *J. Toxicol. Environ. Health.*, 4:107–121.
75. Litterst, C. L., Farber, T. M., Baker, A. M., and VanLoon, E. J. (1972): Effect of polychlorinated biphenyls on hepatic microsomal enzymes in the rat. *Toxicol. Appl. Pharmacol.*, 23:112–122.
76. Lu, A. Y. H., and Levin, W. (1974): The resolution and reconstitution of the liver microsomal hydroxylation system. *Biochem. Biophys. Acta*, 344:205–240.
77. Lu, A. Y. H., Somogyi, A., West, S., Kuntzman, R., and Conney, A. H. (1972): Pregnenolone-16α-carbonitrile: A new type of inducer of drug-metabolizing enzymes. *Arch. Biochem. Biophys.*, 152:457–462.
78. McPherson, F., Bridges, J. W., and Parke, D. V. (1974): *In vitro* enhancement of hepatic microsomal biphenyl 2-hydroxylation by carcinogens. *Nature*, 252:488–489.
79. Mehendale, H. M., Chen, P. R., Fishbein, L., and Matthews, H. B. (1973): Effect of Mirex on the activities of various rat hepatic mixed-function oxidases. *Arch. Environ. Contam. Toxicol.*, 1:245–254.

80. Mehendale, H. M., Takanaka, A., Desaiah, D., and Ho, I. K. (1977): Kepone induction hepatic mixed-function oxidases in the male rat. *Life Sci.*, 20:991–998.

81. Mehendale, H. M., Takanaka, A., Desaiah, D., and Ho, I. K. (1978): Effect of preexposure to Kepone on hepatic mixed-function oxidases in the female rat. *Toxicol. Appl. Pharmacol.*, 44:171–180.

82. Melancon, M. J., Elcombe, C. R., Vodicnik, M. J., and Lech, J. J. (1980): Uptake of microsomal mixed-function oxidase activity in carp (Abstract). *Toxicol. Appl. Pharmacol.*, (*in press*).

83. Melancon, M. J., and Lech, J. J. (1979): Uptake, biotransformation, disposition, and elimination of 2-methylnaphthalene and naphthalene in several fish species. In: *Aquatic Toxicology*, edited by L. L. Marking and R. A. Kimerle, pp. 5–22. American Society for Testing and Materials, Philadelphia.

84. Milnes, D. H. (1971): Formation of 2,3,7,8-tetrachlorodibenzodioxin by thermal decomposition of Na 2,4,5 trichlorophenate. *Nature*, 232:395–396.

85. Nebert, D. W. (1979): Multiple forms of inducible drug-metabolizing enzymes: A reasonable mechanism by which any organism can cope with adversity. *Mol. Cell. Immunol.*, 27:27–46.

86. Payne, J. F. (1976): Field evaluation of benzopyrene hydroxylase induction as a monitor for marine petroleum pollution. *Science*, 191:945–946.

87. Payne, J. F., and May, N. (1979): Further studies on the effect of petroleum hydrocarbons on mixed-function oxidases in marine organisms. In: *Pesticide and Xenobiotic Metabolism in Aquatic Organisms*, edited by M. A. Q. Khan, J. J. Lech, and J. J. Menn, pp. 339–347. American Chemical Society Symposium Series, Washington, D. C.

88. Payne, J. F., and Penrose, W. R. (1975): Induction of aryl hydrocarbon (benzo[a]pyrene) hydroxylase in fish by petroleum. *Bull. Environ. Contam. Toxicol.*, 14:112–116.

89. Pedersen, M. G., Hershberger, W. K., and Juchau, M. R. (1974): Metabolism of 3,4-benzpyrene in rainbow trout. *Bull. Environ. Contam. Toxicol.*, 12:481–486.

90. Pedersen, M. G., Hershberger, W. K., Zachariah, P. K., and Juchau, M. R. (1976): Hepatic biotransformation of environmental xenobiotics in six strains of rainbow trout. *J. Fish Res. Board Can.*, 33:666–675.

91. Platonow, N. S., Kiptrap, R. M., and Geissinger, H. D. (1972): The distribution and excretion of PCBs (Aroclor 1254) and their effect on urinary gonadal steroid levels in the boar. *Bull. Environ. Contam. Toxicol.*, 7:358–365.

92. Pohl, R. J., Bend, J. R., Guarino, A. M., and Fouts, J. R. (1974): Hepatic microsomal mixed-function oxidase activity of several marine species from coastal Maine. *Drug Metab. Dispos.*, 2:454–555.

93. Pohl, R. J., Fouts, J. R., and Bend, J. R. (1975): Response of hepatic microsomal MFO in the little skate and the winter flounder to pretreatment with TCDD or DBA. *Bull. Mount. Desert Biol. Labs*, 15:64–66.

94. Poland, A., and Glover, E. (1977): Chlorinated biphenyl induction of aryl hydrocarbon hydroxylase activity: A study of the structure-activity relationship. *Mol. Pharmacol.*, 13:924–938.

95. Rasmussen, R. E., and Wang, I. Y. (1974): Dependence of specific metabolism of benzo(a)pyrene on the induction of hydroxylase activity. *Cancer Res.*, 34:2,290–2,295.
96. Risebrough, R. W., Reiche, P., Peakall, D. B., Herman, S. G., and Kirven, M. N. (1968): Polychlorinated biphenyls in global ecosystem. *Nature*, 220:1.098–1,102.
97. Schwen, R. (1980): *Phylogenetic Aspects of the Hepatic Cytochrome P-450-Dependent Monooxygenase System.* Ph.D. Thesis, University of Minnesota.
98. Sharma, R. N., Cameron, R. G., Farber, E., Griffin, M. J., Joly, J. G., and Murray, R. K. (1979): Multiplicity of induction patterns of rat liver microsomal monooxygenases and other polypeptides produced by administration of various xenobiotics. *Biochem. J.*, 182:317–327.
99. Sinnhuber, R. O., Hendricks, J. D., Wales, J. H., and Putnam, G. B. (1977): Neoplasms in rainbow trout: A sensitive animal model for environmental carcinogenesis. *Ann. N.Y. Acad. Sci.*, 298:289–408.
100. Sivarajah, K., Franklin, C. S., and Williams, W. P. (1978): The effects of polychlorinated biphenyls on plasma steroid levels and hepatic microsomal enzymes in fish. *J. Fish. Biol.*, 13:401–409.
101. Sladek, W. E., and Mannering, G. J. (1966): Evidence for a new P-450 hemoprotein in hepatic microsomes from methylcholanthrene-treated rats. *Biochem. Biophys. Res. Commun.*, 24:668–674.
102. Snyder, R., and Remmer, H. (1979): Classes of hepatic microsomal mixed-function oxidase inducers. *Pharmacol. Ther.*, 7:203–244.
103. Stanton, R. H., and Khan, M. A. Q. (1975): Components of the mixed-function oxidase system of hepatic microsomes of freshwater fishes. *Gen. Pharmacol.*, 6:289–294.
104. Statham, C. N., Elcombe, C. R., Szyjka, S. P., and Lech, J. J. (1978): Effect of polycyclic aromatic hydrocarbons on hepatic microsomal enzymes and disposition of methylnaphthalene in rainbow trout *in vivo. Xenobiotica*, 8:65–71.
105. Stegeman, J. J. (1977): Fate and effects of oil in marine animals. *Oceanus*, 20:59–66.
106. Stegeman, J. J. (1977): Sex differences in hepatic microsomal cytochrome P-450 in spawning trout (Abstract). *Fed. Proc.*, 36:941.
107. Stegeman, J. J. (1978): Influence of environmental contamination on cytochrome P-450 mixed-function oxygenases in fish: Implications for recovery in the Wild Harbor Marsh. *J. Fish Res. Board Can.*, 35:668–674.
108. Stegeman, J. J. (1979): Temperature influence on basal activity and induction of mixed-function oxygenase activity in *Fundulus heteroclitus. J. Fish Res. Board Can.*, 36:1,400–1,406.
109. Stegeman, J. J., and Binder, R. L. (1979): High benzo(a)pyrene hydroxylase activity in the marine fish, *Stenotomus versicolor. Biochem. Pharmacol.*, 28:1,686–1,688.
110. Stegeman, J. J., and Chevion, M. (1980): Sex differences in cytochrome P-450 and mixed-function oxidase activity in gonadally mature trout. *Biochem. Pharmacol.*, 29:553–558.
111. Stegeman, J. J., and Klotz, A. V. (1979): A possible role for microsomal hexose-6-phosphate dehydrogenase in microsomal electron transport and mixed-function oxidase activity. *Biochem. Biophys. Res. Commun.*, 87:410–415.

112. Stegeman, J. J., and Woodin, B. R. (1980): Patterns of benzo(a)pyrene metabolism in liver of the marine fish *Stenotomus versicolor. Fed. Proc.*, 39:1,752.
113. Stevens, J. T., Chernoff, N., Farmer, J. D., and DiPasquale, L. C. (1979): Perinatal toxicology of Mirex administered in the diet. II. Relationship of hepatic Mirex levels to induction of microsomal benzphetamine-N-demethylase activity. *Toxicol. Lett.*, 4:269–274.
114. Swenson, D. H., Lin, J., Miller, E., and Miller, J. A. (1977): Aflatoxin $B_1$-2,3-oxide as a probable intermediate in the covalent binding of aflatoxins $B_1$ and $B_2$ to rat liver DNA and ribosomal RNA *in vivo. Cancer Res.*, 37:172–181.
115. Thomas, P. E., Lu, A. Y. H., Ryan, D., West, S. B., Kawalek, J., and Levin, W. (1976): Immunochemical evidence for six forms of rat liver cytochrome P-450 and P-448. *Mol. Pharmacol.*, 12:746–758.
116. Tucker, A. N., and Tang, T. (1979): Effects of phenobarbital and methylcholanthrene on hepatic mixed-function oxidase activities in hamsters. *J. Environ. Pathol. Toxicol.*, 2:613–623.
117. Uehleke, H. (1967): Stimulurung einiger mikrosomaler Frendstoff-Oxydationen durch Phenobarbital, Methylcholanthren, and Chlorophenathan, einzeln und in Kombination. *Naunyn-Schmiedebergs Arch. Pharmak. U. Exp. Path.*, 259:66–90.
118. Vainio, H. (1974): Enhancement of hepatic microsomal drug oxidation and glucuronidation in rat by 1,1,1-trichloro-2,2-bis (*p*-chlorophenyl) ethane (DDT). *Chem. Biol. Interact.*, 9:7–14.
119. Vainio, H., and Hanninen, O. (1974): A comparative study on drug hydroxylation and glucuronidation in liver microsomes of phenobarbital and 3-methylcholanthrene treated rats. *Acta Pharmacol. Toxicol.*, 35:65–75.
120. Varanasi, V., and Gmur, D. (1980): Metabolic activation and covalent binding of benzo(a)pyrene to deoxyribonucleic acid catalyzed by liver enzymes of marine fish. *Biochem. Pharmacol.*, 29:753–761.
121. Vodicnik, M. J., Elcombe, C. R., and Lech, J. J. (1980): The effect of sex steroids and pregnenolone-16α-carbonitrile on hepatic monooxygenase activity in the rainbow trout. *Toxicol. Appl. Pharmacol. (Abstr.)*53:A118.
122. Vodicnik, M. J., Elcombe, C. R., and Lech, J. J. (1981): The effect of various types of inducing agents on hepatic microsomal monooxygenase activity in rainbow trout. *Toxicol. Appl. Pharmacol.* 59:364–374.
123. Walton, D. G., Dawe, L. L., Green, J. M., Kiceniuk, J. W., May, N., Murphy, R. G., Penrose, W. R., and White, M. D. (1980): Effects of captivity and petroleum exposure on the reproductive cycle of the cunner. *Mar. Sci. Res. Lab. Contribution #366*, Dept. Fish. Oceans, St. Johns, Newfoundland.
124. Walton, D. G., Penrose, W. R., and Green, J. M. (1978): The petroleum-inducible mixed-function oxidase of cunner; Some characteristics relevant to hydrocarbon monitoring. *J. Fish Res. Board Can.*, 35:1,547–1,552.
125. Welton, A. F., and Aust, S. D. (1974): The effects of 3-methylcholanthrene and phenobarbital induction on the structure of rat liver endoplasmic reticulum. *Biochem. Biophys. Acta*, 373:197–210.

*Aquatic Toxicology*, edited by Lavern J. Weber.
Raven Press, New York © 1982.

# Chemical Carcinogenesis in Fish

## Jerry D. Hendricks

*Department of Food Science and Technology, Oregon State University,
Corvallis, Oregon 97331*

Spontaneous neoplasms in fish, both as isolated and epizootic occurrences, have been reported by numerous authors. The subject has been extensively reviewed (15,16,63,64,114) and will not be further discussed at this time. Spontaneous epizootics of fish cancer, especially the aflatoxin-induced rainbow trout (*Salmo gairdneri*) liver cancer outbreak of the early 1960s (73), have served as the stimulus for subsequent studies on experimental, chemically induced carcinogenesis in fish. Again, the numerous initial experimental studies investigating the etiology of trout liver cancer have been thoroughly reviewed (4,5,27,28) and will not be discussed in this review.

Subsequent to the early trout hepatoma work, chemically induced carcinogenesis studies in fish have developed along two primary lines: (a) the use of rainbow trout as experimental animals to further elucidate the metabolism and carcinogenicity of aflatoxin $B_1$ ($AFB_1$) and its metabolites, as well as other chemical carcinogens (85), and (b) the use of various small aquarium fish species as rapid whole-animal model systems to test the carcinogenicity of suspect chemicals (62). Interest in fish oncology results not only from the comparative point of view with possible benefits to the fishery profession but also from the human health standpoint, since fish may be sensitive first-line indicators of environmental contamination which could have important public health significance.

*149*

## CHEMICAL CARCINOGENESIS IN SALMONIDS

### Introduction

Most of the research on experimental carcinogenesis in salmonids has been conducted by two research groups. Early studies into the etiology of the trout liver cancer epizootic were performed at the U.S. Fish and Wildlife Service's Western Fish Nutrition Laboratory at Cook, Washington, under the direction of Drs. John E. Halver and Laurence M. Ashley. A continuing study of the metabolism and carcinogenicity of $AFB_1$ and its metabolites in rainbow trout, as well as the development of the rainbow trout as a documented research animal for carcinogenic and toxicologic research, has occurred for the past 16 years at the Food Toxicology and Nutrition Laboratory (FTNL) in the Department of Food Science and Technology at Oregon State University under the direction of Professor Russell O. Sinnhuber.

With few exceptions, to be noted later, carcinogenicity studies in salmonids to date have centered around liver carcinogenesis. This is to be expected, since the focus has been on powerful liver carcinogens, i.e., aflatoxins and nitrosamines. As a result, very little is known about the metabolism of and the response to other organ-specific carcinogens of salmonids.

Since fish experimental carcinogenesis is still basically an infant discipline, an extensive framework of basic physiologic, biochemical, nutritional, and clinical information is not available, as is the case in rodent experimental carcinogenesis. Therefore, many of the experiments that have been conducted thus far have had a dual purpose. First, there has been the desire to derive biomedically significant data from the use of aquatic species. Second, and perhaps just as important, has been the desire and need to establish baseline information to define the aquatic model systems as completely as possible.

## Species Sensitivity

Rainbow trout, *Salmo gairdneri*, members of the teleost fish family Salmonidae (the salmon, trout, and char), are more sensitive to aflatoxin carcinogenicity than are any other known group of animals or species of fish (51,109,117). Many of the species, subspecies, and strains of salmon, trout, and char have been tested intentionally or unintentionally for their sensitivity to aflatoxin. The Shasta strain, maintained as an outbred population at the FTNL, appears to be the most sensitive of the various genetic strains of rainbow trout, including the Kamloops, Donaldson, and wild steelhead strains (85,88,109,117). Liver cancer has been produced in brook trout, *Salvelinus fontinalis*, but the sensitivity was significantly lower than rainbow trout (118). Brown trout (*Salmo trutta*) also were much less susceptible to $AFB_1$ than rainbow trout (109). The Pacific salmon (Genus *Oncorhynchus*) are relatively insensitive to aflatoxins. Wolf and Jackson (118) failed to induce liver tumors in coho salmon (*O. kisutch*) with $AFB_1$. Wales and Sinnhuber (111) were able to produce tumors in sockeye salmon (*O. nerka*) only by feeding $AFB_1$ plus cyclopropenoid fatty acids, synergists that promote $AFB_1$ carcinogenicity. We have been able to induce tumors in coho salmon by embryo exposure with $AFB_1$, but the incidence was much lower than comparably exposed rainbow trout (J. D. Hendricks, *unpublished data*). Efforts to produce an inbred strain from the outbred Shasta strain, selected for extreme $AFB_1$ sensitivity, have not been attempted, but it is conceivable that the high sensitivity of Shasta rainbows could be further increased in this way. Even though Shasta rainbow trout are extremely sensitive to liver carcinogenesis, spontaneous liver neoplasms are rare in trout fed the control diet for 1 year. This feature enhances their value as research animals for carcinogenesis, since any neoplasms observed in trout on experimental diets can normally be attributed to the suspect chemical.

## Routes of Exposure

### Dietary

At the FTNL, as at other reseach centers using salmonids as experimental animals for cancer research, the primary route of exposure to chemical carcinogens has been dietary. This has been facilitated by the development and use of a semipurified test diet, the Oregon Test Diet (OTD), (85,90) the formula of which is shown in Table 1. Nonpolar, lipid-soluble carcinogens can be added easily to the fish oil fraction, thoroughly mixed, and then incorporated

TABLE 1. *Oregon Test Diet*

| Ingredient | Percent |
|---|---|
| Casein | 49.5 |
| Gelatin | 8.7 |
| Dextrin | 15.6 |
| Mineral mix[a] | 4.0 |
| Carboxymethyl cellulose[b] | 1.0 |
| $\alpha$-cellulose | 8.2 |
| Choline-chloride (70%) | 1.0 |
| Vitamin mix[c] | 2.0 |
| Fish oil (salmon or herring) | 10.0 |

[a]Calcium carbonate ($CaCO_3$, 2.100%), calcium phosphate ($CaHPO_4 \cdot 2H_2O$, 73.500%), potassium phosphate ($K_2HPO_4$, 8.100%), potassium sulfate ($K_2SO_4$, 6.800%), sodium chloride (NaCl, 3.060%), sodium phosphate ($Na_2HPO_4 \cdot 6H_2O$, 2.140%), magnesium oxide (MgO, 2.500%), ferric citrate ($FeC_6H_5O_7 \cdot 3H_2O$, 0.558%), manganese carbonate ($MnCO_3$, 0.418%), cupric carbonate ($2CuCO_3Cu(OH)_2$, 0.034%), zinc carbonate ($ZnCO_3$, 0.081%), potassium iodide (KI, 0.001%), sodium fluoride (NaF, 0.002%), cobalt chloride ($CoCl_2$, 0.020%), and citric acid ($C_6H_8O_7 \cdot H_2O$, 0.686%).

[b]Hercules Powder Company, San Francisco, California.

[c]Thiamine hydrochloride (0.3200%), riboflavin (0.7200%), niacinamide (2.5600%), biotin (0.0080%), D-calcium pantothenate (1.4400%), pyridoxine hydrochloride (0.2400%), folic acid (0.0960%), menadione (0.0800%), vitamin $B_{12}$ (cobalamine, 3000 $\mu$g/g, 0.2667%), *i*-inositol (*meso*, 12.5000%), ascorbic acid (6.0000%), *p*-aminobenzoic acid (2.0000%), vitamin $D_3$ (1,000,000 USP/g, 0.0050%), vitamin A (250,000 units/g, 0.5000%), *dl-a*-tocopherol (250 IU/g, 13.2%), and $\alpha$-cellulose (60.0643%).

From Sinnhuber et al. (85).

into the remainder of the diet by the following procedure. Hot water (55 to 60°C) is added to the dry ingredients; the toxin-containing lipid is then added and thoroughly mixed with an electric stirrer. Final water content is 65%, and cooling in a cold water bath produces an easily handled, solid, gel-like diet. It can then be cut into appropriate sizes with slicers and dicers and fed to fish fresh, or frozen for future use. Polar compounds can also be readily added in the water and mixed into the diet. This diet produces rapid growth, normal sexual maturation and viability, and normal tissue histology in rainbow trout, and recently has been used for a number of other freshwater and marine teleosts and crustaceans. Dry food conversion in the Shasta strain rainbow trout, at a constant water temperature of 12°C, varies between 0.7 and 1.2 (dry food consumed per wet weight gained), depending on fish age.

Most dietary carcinogen exposures at the FTNL have involved the continuous feeding of specified levels of carcinogen throughout the duration of the trial, usually 12 months. On occasion, carcinogens have been fed for 12 months, and the fish have been maintained on the control diet for an additional 3 to 6 months to permit full tumor expression. It is probably not necessary to feed rainbow trout the entire 12 months, during a 12-month trial, to produce the maximum tumor expression at 12 months. It is highly probable that the final few months of carcinogen feeding contribute little, if any, to the final tumor incidence, since a definite latent period, from tumor initiation to tumor expression, is involved. The details of this optimum feeding period remain to be established. Recently, short-term (2 to 4 weeks) dietary exposures to relatively high $AFB_1$ doses (10 to 20 ppb) have proved effective for inducing high incidences of liver cancer. The short-term exposures also provide greater flexibility for studying the effects of induction and/or promotion on experimental carcinogenesis. Both long- and short-term feeding trials with levels of 4 ppb or above tend to produce rainbow trout livers with multiple tumors, often 10 or more. Low dietary levels tend to produce fewer tumors per liver as well as fewer tumor-bearing animals.

## *Embryo*

A second exposure route for carcinogens in trout and other teleosts is the static exposure of fertile embryos (eggs) to a solution of the carcinogen (31,32,34–37,110,113). A routine exposure procedure at the FTNL includes the following: 200 21-day-old rainbow trout eggs (hatching occurs 24 days postfertilization at 12°C) are placed into a 200 ml solution of carcinogen for 0.5 to 1.0 hr (maintained at 12°C with water bath), rinsed in fresh water several times, and returned to incubator compartment for hatching. Following hatching and yolk sac absorption, the fry are fed the OTD for 12 months and examined grossly and histopathologically for tumor development. Depending on the conditions, this exposure is highly effective and requires significantly less chemical to produce a given tumor incidence response than with dietary exposures (113). It has the added advantages of more uniform exposure of the carcinogen to each individual animal, single as opposed to multiple carcinogen handlings by personnel, and ease of carcinogen containment and decontamination. It is interesting that embryo exposure to carcinogens tends to produce livers with usually one and rarely more than three to four tumors per liver, in contrast to dietary exposure which usually produces multiple tumors, even though the two exposures may produce the same number of tumor-bearing animals. This may be the result of single as opposed to continuous exposure and the subsequent effects of DNA repair. More specifics about this technique will be given later in this review.

## *Injection and Gavage*

Other less commonly employed routes of exposure used with salmonids include i.p. injections (79) and stomach gavage (45). The latter appears to present particular difficulties with some fish species since regurgitation (especially with rainbow trout) is very common.

## Carcinogenicity of Chemicals to Rainbow Trout

The total number of proven carcinogens in rainbow trout is still relatively few compared with mammalian species, simply because few have been tested. They can be placed in four general classes as follows: (a) mycotoxins, (b) cyclopropenoid fatty acids, (c) nitrosamines, and (d) miscellaneous. A review of the available information on the metabolism and carcinogenicity of compounds in each of these groups will now be presented.

*Mycotoxins*

Naturally occurring aflatoxins ($AFB_1$, $AFG_1$, $AFB_2$, $AFG_2$) are shown in Fig. 1.

*Carcinogenicity*

The aforementioned epizootic of liver cancer in hatchery-reared rainbow trout provided the stimulus for extensive research on the metabolism and carcinogenicity of $AFB_1$ in mammalian species as well as rainbow trout. The high incidence and severity of liver cancer in this epizootic provided initial evidence that the rainbow trout was extremely sensitive to $AFB_1$. Subsequent feeding trials (51,86,89) demonstrated that dietary levels in the low ppb range (4 to 8 ppb) were adequate to produce a significant incidence of liver cancer in rainbow trout in 1 year. Lee et al. (51) also showed that continuous feeding of $AFB_1$ at levels as low as 0.4 ppb would still elicit a carcinogenic response (Table 2). Lee et al. (53) observed that higher dietary levels for short periods of time, as little as 1 day, were also effective in inducing liver tumors (Table 3). Thus, extremely small amounts of aflatoxin are required to elicit a neoplastic response in rainbow trout. In general, the sensitivity of our FTNL Shasta strain rainbow trout to $AFB_1$ has increased over the past 16 years and may be attributable to either some degree of unintentional inbreeding or improvements that have been made in the Oregon Test Diet. We have seen a definite relationship between nutritional state of the trout and its susceptibility to tumor development. Vigorous, fast-growing trout are usually more susceptible to tumor initiation and growth than stunted, slow-growing trout. Thus, nutritional improvements may encourage tumor growth as well as body growth.

Early experimentation with the embryo exposure technique of tumor initiation in rainbow trout utilized $AFB_1$ as the model car-

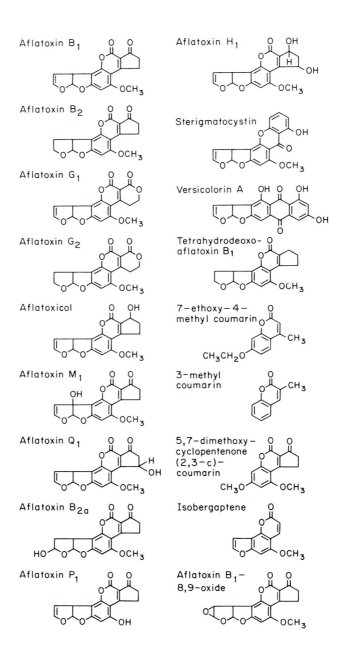

Aflatoxin B₁

Aflatoxin H₁

Aflatoxin B₂

Sterigmatocystin

Aflatoxin G₁

Versicolorin A

Aflatoxin G₂

Tetrahydrodeoxo-aflatoxin B₁

Aflatoxicol

7-ethoxy-4-methyl coumarin

Aflatoxin M₁

3-methyl coumarin

Aflatoxin Q₁

5,7-dimethoxy-cyclopentenone (2,3-c)-coumarin

Aflatoxin B₂ₐ

Isobergaptene

Aflatoxin P₁

Aflatoxin B₁-8,9-oxide

**FIG. 1.**   Chemical structures of mycotoxins and related compounds.

TABLE 2. *Liver tumor incidence in rainbow trout fed carcinogenic diets with and without CPFAs*

| | | Hepatoma | Incidence[a] |
|---|---|---|---|
| Diet no. | Diet description | No. | % |
| 12 months[b] | | | |
| 1 | Control | 0/50 | 0 |
| 2 | Control + 4 ppb AFB₁ | 10/20 | 50 |
| 3 | Control + 0.02% *Sterculia foetida* oil[c] | 12/116 | 10 |
| 4 | Control + 0.02% *Sterculia foetida* oil + 4 ppb AFB₁ | 57/58 | 98 |
| 5 | Control + 0.01% *Sterculia foetida* oil | 1/136 | 0.7 |
| 6 | Control + 0.01% *Sterculia foetida* oil + 4 ppb AFB₁ | 112/112 | 100 |
| 7 | Control + 0.10% *Hibiscus syriacus* oil[d] | 5/133 | 3.7 |
| 8 | Control + 0.10% *Hibiscus syriacus* oil + 4 ppb AFB₁ | 119/119 | 100 |
| 9 | Control + 0.10% *Hibiscus syriacus* oil + 200 ppm gossypol + 4 ppb AFB₁ | 117/119 | 98 |
| 15 months | | | |
| 1 | Control | 0/50 | 0 |
| 2 | Control + 4 ppb AFB₁ | 65/108 | 60 |
| 10 | Control + 0.4 ppb AFB₁ | 15/106 | 14 |
| 11 | Control + 0.10% *Hibiscus syriacus* oil + 0.4 ppb AFB₁ | 42/105 | 40 |
| 12 | Control + 100 ppm acetylaminofluorene | 0/95 | 0 |
| 13 | Control + 0.10% *Hibiscus syriacus* oil + 100 ppm 2-acetylaminofluorene | 20/102 | 20 |

[a]Results are expressed as number of trout with tumors/total number of trout.
[b]Experiments 3 through 9 were terminated at 9-1/2 months.
[c]*Sterculia foetida* oil contained 49% sterculic and 7% malvalic acids.
[d]*Hibiscus syriacus* oil contained 19% malvalic and 2% sterculic acids.
From Lee et al. (51).

TABLE 3. *The effect of methyl sterculate on the initiation of trout liver tumors by 20 ppb AFB,*

| Group | Time on toxic diets (days) | AFB, consumed (μg/kg body weight) | Sterculate consumed (mg/kg body weight) | 12-mo. tumor incidence No. | % | Average no. of nodes/liver | Average tumor volume (cu mm) |
|---|---|---|---|---|---|---|---|
| 1 | 1 | 0.55 | 0 | 2/59 | 3.4 | 0.03 (1.0)[a] | 17.0 |
| 2 | 5 | 1.73 | 0 | 6/51 | 11.7 | 0.26 (2.2) | 17.6 |
| 3 | 10 | 3.25 | 0 | 5/50 | 10.0 | 0.10 (1.0) | 0.9 |
| 4 | 20 | 6.98 | 0 | 23/57 | 40.3 | 0.95 (2.4) | 2.2 |
| 5 | 30 | 10.31 | 0 | 17/47 | 36.1 | 0.97 (2.6) | 1.0 |
| 6 | 1 | 0.51 | 2.55 | 0/45 | 0 | | |
| 7 | 5 | 1.81 | 9.05 | 9/53 | 16.9 | 0.23 (1.3) | 19.2 |
| 8 | 10 | 3.32 | 16.60 | 16/60 | 26.6 | 0.45 (1.7) | 2.2 |
| 9 | 20 | 6.42 | 32.10 | 42/57 | 73.6 | 3.10 (5.4) | 17.2 |
| 10 | 30 | 9.18 | 45.90 | 23/27 | 85.2 | 6.15 (7.2) | 19.6 |

[a]Number in parentheses = number of tumors/liver if only livers with hepatoma are considered.
From Lee et al. (53).

cinogen. These studies showed that a brief exposure of trout eggs to a weak solution (0.5 ppm) of $AFB_1$ was sufficient to initiate a significant incidence of hepatocellular carcinomas, grossly evident 6 to 12 months later (113). These studies also established that a 1.0 ppm solution of $AFB_1$ for a 1-hr exposure was lethal to all the embryos and that a 2-hr exposure at 0.5 ppm did not significantly increase the tumor incidence over a 1-hr exposure (45% versus 42%, respectively) (113). Acute effects of $AFB_1$ exposure to embryos were found in both liver and kidney tissue. Slight to severe liver necrosis occurred following exposure to 0.5 ppm $AFB_1$ for 1 hr, but mortalities appeared to result primarily from kidney necrosis and renal failure, since moribund fry always presented a severe ascitic condition (113). The sensitivity of rainbow trout embryos to $AFB_1$ carcinogenesis was found to increase with age during the developmental period, with greatest sensitivity just before hatching (113) (Table 4). Additional water exposures with hatched sac-fry showed further increased sensitivity to $AFB_1$ carcinogenicity and

TABLE 4. *Hepatocellular carcinoma incidence in rainbow trout treated on alternate days during embryonic development in 0.5 ppm AFB$_1$ for 1 hr*

| Age of embryo (days) | 10-month incidence[a] (%) | 12-month incidence[a] (%) | Total no. of tumors | No. of tumors/liver[b] | Average tumor diameter (mm)[b] |
|---|---|---|---|---|---|
| 1 | 0/25 (0.0) | 0/59 (0.0) | 0 | 0 | 0.0 |
| 3 | – (–) | 2/53 (3.8) | 2 | 1.0 ± 0 (2) | 3.0 ± 0 (2) |
| 5 | 4/48 (8.3) | 11/58 (19.0) | 14 | 1.3 ± 0.5 (11) | 5.3 ± 4.8 (14) |
| 7 | 3/39 (7.7) | 11/55 (20.0) | 12 | 1.1 ± 0.3 (11) | 2.9 ± 1.2 (12) |
| 9 | 5/35 (14.3) | 11/62 (17.7) | 11 | 1.2 ± 0.6 (11) | 3.4 ± 2.3 (13) |
| 11 | 4/30 (13.3) | 11/60 (18.3) | 13 | 1.2 ± 0.4 (11) | 4.2 ± 3.6 (13) |
| 13 | 1/45 (2.2) | 10/60 (16.7) | 13 | 1.3 ± 0.5 (10) | 3.2 ± 1.6 (13) |
| 15 | 11/52 (21.2) | 19/60 (31.7) | 29 | 1.5 ± 0.8 (19) | 4.1 ± 3.5 (29) |
| 17 | 13/39 (33.3) | 29/63 (46.0) | 46 | 1.6 ± 1.4 (29) | 4.2 ± 2.2 (46) |
| 19 | 18/42 (42.9) | 29/59 (49.2) | 42 | 1.4 ± 0.9 (29) | 6.2 ± 4.6 (42) |
| 21 | 20/36 (55.5) | 33/55 (60.0) | 48 | 1.5 ± 0.9 (33) | 4.2 ± 2.8 (48) |
| 23 | 20/35 (57.1) | 35/60 (58.3) | 48 | 1.4 ± 0.6 (35) | 6.6 ± 4.4 (48) |
| Control | 0/40 (0.0) | 0/60 (0.0) | 0 | 0 | 0.0 |

[a]Number of trout with tumors/total number of trout. Dash indicates no sample taken.
[b]Values are expressed as means ± SD; numbers in parentheses indicate the number of samples.

From Wales et al. (113).

lethality with increased age during the yolk sac stage, and maximum carcinogenic sensitivity at the swimup stage about 2.5 weeks post-hatching (37) (Table 5). Since $AFB_1$ requires metabolic activation by the liver, as will be discussed later, this increased sensitivity to $AFB_1$ with increased age is probably partially due to the rapidly increasing mass of liver tissue in the older embryos/fish and also possibly to greater enzymatic activity in the liver of the older in-dividuals. Wales et al. (113) demonstrated the uptake of $AFB_1$ into trout embryos after exposure of embryos to $[^{14}C]AFB_1$ (Table 6). The absence of the protective egg chorion may permit more $AFB_1$ uptake by the hatched sac-fry, resulting in the greater lethal and carcinogenic response seen (37).

Subsequent embryo exposure experiments were focused at max-imizing the response of embryos to $AFB_1$ and included exposures

TABLE 5. *Increased sensitivity of rainbow trout (embryos/sac-fry) to the lethal and carcinogenic effects of $AFB_1$ treatment[a]*

| Age[b] | Treatment | Cumulative 90-day mortality | Liver tumor incidence[c] 12 months | % |
|---|---|---|---|---|
| 14[d] | $AFB_1$ | 27 | 57/119 | 48 |
| | Sham | 18 | 1/118 | 0.8 |
| 21[d] | $AFB_1$ | 39 | 79/120 | 66 |
| | Sham | 41 | 0/107 | 0 |
| 28[e] | $AFB_1$ | 265 | 56/102 | 55 |
| | Sham | 25 | 0/120 | 0 |
| 35[e] | $AFB_1$ | 144 | 38/58 | 66 |
| 42[f] | $AFB_1$ | 157 | 40/45 | 88 |
| | Sham | 3 | 0/120 | 0 |

[a]Treatment was 0.5 ppm $AFB_1$ for 1 hr; age of embryos/sac-fry increased from 14 days postfertilization to yolk sac resorption.
[b]Age of embryos or sac-fry, in days postfertilization.
[c]Results expressed as number of trout with tumors/total num-ber of trout.
[d]Eyed-egg stage.
[e]Hatching complete, sac-fry stage.
[f]Yolk sac absorbed, fry stage.
From Hendricks et al. (37).

TABLE 6. *[¹⁴C] content of rainbow trout eggs and sac-fry as a function of time after treatment of 21-day eggs with [¹⁴C]AFB₁*

| Time after treatment | [¹⁴C]AFB₁ ng/egg or sac-fry[a] |
|---|---|
| | Eggs |
| 30 min | 29.9 ± 6.0 (6,2) |
| 1 day | 3.8 ± 0.5 (6,2) |
| 2 days | 3.3 ± 0.4 (2,3) |
| 3 days | 3.3 ± 0.9 (8,2) |
| 4 days | 3.2 ± 0.5 (6,2) |
| | Sac-fry |
| 7 days | 1.6 ± 0.6 (12,2) |
| 8 days | 1.8 ± 0.5 (6,2) |
| 9 days | 1.5 ± 0.4 (6,2) |
| 10 days | 1.4 ± 0.2 (6,4) |
| 11 days | 1.6 ± 0.2 (6,5) |

[a]Values are means ± SD expressed as ng [¹⁴C]AFB₁ per egg or sac-fry assuming ¹⁴C is in AFB₁ and a specific activity of 0.037 $\mu$C/$\mu$g AFB₁. First number in the parenthesis is the number of samples; second number is the number of eggs or sac-fry in each sample.
From Wales et al. (113).

to determine the effect of dose (Table 7) and length of exposure (Table 8) on tumor expression (37). These data have resulted in the development of a standard procedure for rainbow trout embryo exposure to AFB₁: 21-day-old embryos (to maximize sensitivity but avoid early hatching individuals) are exposed to a 0.5 ppm solution (to maximize carcinogenic, but minimize lethal, insult) for 30 min (the length of time giving maximum tumor response). This exposure method routinely results in 65 to 70% of the exposed fish developing one or more grossly observable liver carcinomas at 12 months (37).

To my knowledge, there has been only one published report of rainbow trout exposure to AFB₁ by i.p. injection. Scarpelli (79) exposed rainbow trout fingerlings to twice weekly injections of 0.06 mg AFB₁/kg body weight in propylene glycol for 25 weeks for a

TABLE 7. *Effect of AFB₁-concentration on the hepatocellular carcinoma incidence in rainbow trout treated for 1 hr as 21-day-old embryos*

| Concentration | Hepatocellular carcinoma incidence[a] | | | |
|---|---|---|---|---|
| of AFB$_1$ (ppm) | 9 months | % | 12 months | % |
| 0.05 | 9/81 | 11 | 32/120 | 27 |
| 0.1 | 16/76 | 21 | 58/118 | 49 |
| 0.2 | 31/83 | 37 | 74/119 | 62 |
| 0.5 | 21/62 | 34 | 79/120 | 66 |
| Control[b] | 0/65 | 0 | 0/107 | 0 |

[a]Results are expressed as number of trout with tumors/total number of trout.
[b]Well-water sham.
From Hendricks et al. (37).

TABLE 8. *Effects of length of exposure time on carcinogenic response in trout exposed to 0.5 ppm AFB₁ as 21-day-old embryos*

| Exposure | Hepatocellular carcinoma incidences[a] | | | |
|---|---|---|---|---|
| time (min) | 9 months | % | 12 months | % |
| 15 | 14/79 | 19 | 58/119 | 49 |
| 30 | 37/85 | 44 | 86/118 | 73 |
| 60 | 21/62 | 34 | 79/120 | 66 |
| Control | 0/65 | 0 | 0/107 | 0 |

[a]Results expressed as number of trout with tumors/total number of trout.
From Hendricks et al. (37).

total dose of 2.5 mg AFB$_1$/kg body weight. After 50 weeks, 16 of 20 trout had liver tumors. Scarpelli (79) also injected another group of trout with 5 mg SKF-525A [a mixed-function oxidase (MFO) inhibitor]/kg body weight 3 hr prior to each AFB$_1$ injection to demonstrate the importance of MFO activation of AFB$_1$. After 50 weeks, only 1 of 17 of these trout had liver tumors, showing the necessity of AFB$_1$ activation by the MFO system.

Although $AFB_1$ is the most carcinogenic naturally occurring aflatoxin, aflatoxin $G_1$ ($AFG_1$) is also a potent liver carcinogen. Ayres et al. (9) showed that $AFG_1$ was much less carcinogenic to rainbow trout than $AFB_1$ (Table 9), even though it possesses the same terminal double bond on the bifuran rings. Thus, substitution of the cyclopentenone ring on $AFB_1$ by the di-lactone ring of $AFG_1$ markedly reduces the carcinogenicity of $AFG_1$. These authors also failed to produce tumors with the saturated counterparts of $AFB_1$ and $AFG_1$, $AFB_2$ and $AFG_2$, and other compounds with structural similarities to portions of the $AFB_1$ molecule. $AFB_2$, however, fed together with $AFB_1$, exerted a synergistic effect on the carcinogenicity of $AFB_1$ (Table 9), and Wogan et al. (115) produced hepatic tumors in rats with high doses of $AFB_2$. They suggested that $AFB_2$ was converted to $AFB_1$ *in vivo* before it was carcinogenic. Thus, the double bond on the bifuran ring structure appears essential to the carcinogenicity of the aflatoxins, but other modifications on the molecule also severely change the carcinogenicity.

TABLE 9. *Liver tumor incidence in trout fed test diets*

| Diet description | 12 months Number[a] | Percent | 16 months Number[a] | Percent |
|---|---|---|---|---|
| Control | 0/20 | 0 | 0/40 | 0 |
| 4 ppb AFB₁ | 10/40 | 25 | 14/40 | 35 |
| 8 ppb AFB₁ | 40/57 | 70 | 32/40 | 80 |
| 4 ppb AFB₁ + 4 ppb AFB₂ | 17/40 | 43 | 28/40 | 70 |
| 20 ppb AFB₁ | 62/80 | 78 | — | — |
| 20 ppb AFB₂ | 1/20 | 5 | 0/40 | 0 |
| 20 ppb AFG₁ | 1/20 | 5 | 7/40 | 17 |
| 20 ppb AFG₂ | 0/20 | 0 | 0/40 | 0 |
| 20 ppb 7-ethoxy-4-methylcoumarin | 0/40 | 0 | — | — |
| 20 ppb isobergaptene | 0/80 | 0 | — | — |
| 20 ppb tetrahydrodeoxo-AFB₁ | 1/80 | 1 | — | — |
| 20 ppb 5,7-dimethoxycyclopentenone (2,3-c)-coumarin | 0/80 | 0 | — | — |

[a]Results expressed as number of trout with tumors/total number of trout. From Ayres et al. (9).

Data from the exposure of 21-day-old rainbow trout embryos to AFG$_1$ also demonstrates the reduced carcinogenicity of AFG$_1$ relative to AFB$_1$ (Table 10) (37).

*Pathogenesis*

The pathogenesis of AFB$_1$-induced hepatic tumors in rainbow trout has not been thoroughly investigated. It appears, however, that the trout does not present the multiple preneoplastic stages that have been described for rat hepatocarcinogenesis (92,94). Sinnhuber et al. (85) summarized the morphologic stages observed in rainbow trout liver carcinogenesis as follows: (a) diffuse, pale, swollen hepatocytes with enlarged pleomorphic nuclei, (b) eosinophilic foci, (c) basophilic foci, (d) basophilic nodules, and (e) hepatocellular carcinomas.

The cells of the first group (Fig. 2a and b) appear degenerate and do not form proliferating nodules. They result from the toxic properties of AFB$_1$ that apparently interfere with normal cell functions and division, resulting in a polyploid megalocyte that eventually degenerates and becomes necrotic. The eosinophilic cells of the second category are enlarged, glycogen-depleted hepatocytes that often show mitoses and assume nodular arrangements (Fig. 2c). They are almost always infiltrated and sequestered into isolated

TABLE 10. *Hepatocarcinogenicity of AFB$_1$ and its metabolites in rainbow trout exposed as embryos*

| Metabolite tested | Age of embryos | Length of exposure | Concentration of exposure solution | Liver cancer incidence[a] 12 months | 15 months |
|---|---|---|---|---|---|
| AFB$_1$ | 14 | 1 hr | 0.5 ppm | 53/100 | — |
| AFL | 14 | 1 hr | 0.5 ppm | 58/100 | — |
| AFM$_1$ | 21 | 30 min | 5.0 ppm | 0/30 | 1/32 |
| AFO$_1$ | 14 | 1 hr | 1.0 ppm | 0/200 | — |
| AFB$_{2a}$ | 14 | 1 hr | 4.5 ppm | 0/100 | — |
| AFG$_1$ | 21 | 30 min | 5.0 ppm | 2/30 | 7/30 |

[a]Results expressed as number of trout with tumors/total number of trout. From Hendricks et al. (37).

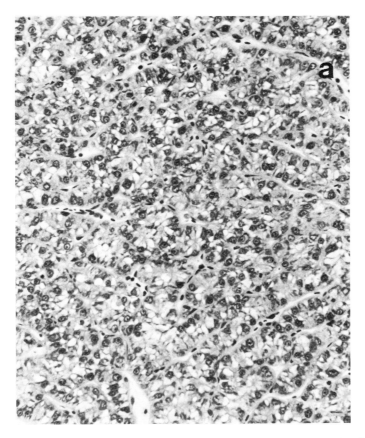

**FIG. 2a.** A section of control rainbow trout liver from a fish fed the OTD for 12 months. Hepatocytes are arranged in cords or tubules two cells in width. Vacuoles are the result of glycogen storage. Nuclei are uniform in size and shape. Hematoxylin and eosin, × 512.

groups of degenerating cells by lymphocytes, however, so it is doubtful if they contribute significantly to the carcinogenic process. The third category, basophilic foci, are commonly seen in trout livers 4 to 6 months after $AFB_1$ exposure (Fig. 2d). They consist of small collections of unencapsulated, basophilic, glycogen-deficient cells with slightly enlarged vesicular nuclei. They may occur

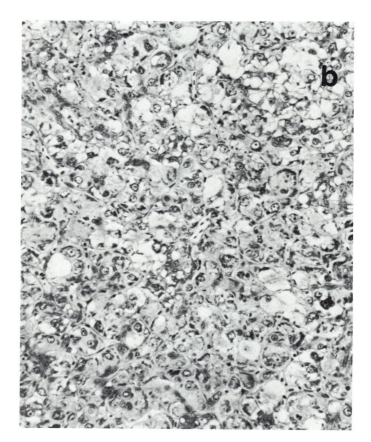

**FIG. 2b:**   Liver tissue from a rainbow trout fed 54 ppb AFB₁ for 6 months. Note the hypertrophied, degenerate cells, with enlarged, often hyperchromatic nuclei. Normal hepatic architecture has been destroyed and several cells have become necrotic and sloughed. Small foci of basophilic regenerating cells are also visible. Hematoxylin and eosin, × 512.

in hepatic cords/tubules of normal two-cell width or in widened cords of three or more cells. Increased mitotic activity is usually obvious, but no compression of surrounding normal tissue occurs. These cells usually occur in the midst of normal appearing hepatocytes with no evidence of prior preneoplastic stages. They rarely

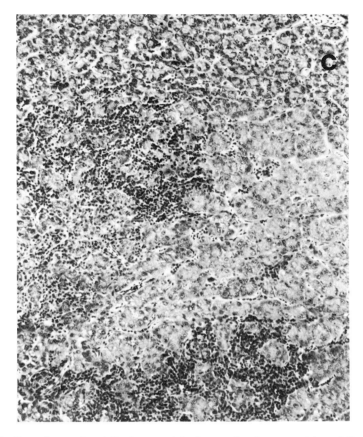

**FIG. 2c.** An eosinophilic liver nodule from a trout exposed to a 0.5 ppm solution of AFB₁ as an embryo. Note the small, normal liver parenchymal cells (*top*), the enlarged eosinophilic cells (*right and center*), and the invading lymphocytes (*center and bottom*). Eosinophilic cells have been sequestered at both sites of lymphocytic invasion. Hematoxylin and eosin, × 320. (From Sinnhuber et al., ref. 85.)

elicit an immune (lymphocytic) response (112) and the cells appear very similar to those found in trabecular hepatocellular carcinomas. Occasionally larger nodules of basophilic cells that are clearly not carcinomas are observed in carcinogen-exposed fish livers. The cells of these nodules are essentially normal, with the exception of a

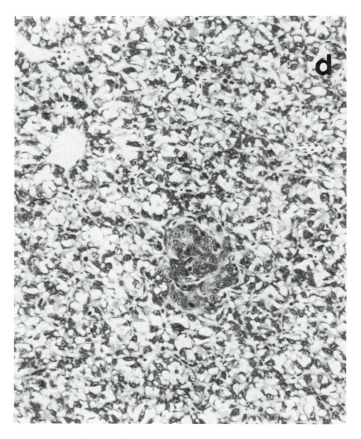

**FIG. 2d.** A small focus of basophilic cells in the midst of essentially normal, glycogen-laden parenchymal cells. This trout had been fed a diet containing 6 ppb $AFB_1$ for 6 months. Note the distinct basophilia, mitotic figure, and slightly enlarged, vesicular nuclei. Hematoxylin and eosin, $\times$ 512. (From Sinnhuber et al., ref. 85.)

definite basophilic staining characteristic (Fig. 3a). The cells are generally normal in size, occur in cords/tubules that are usually two cells in width, usually have some degree of glycogen storage, few mitoses, and normal appearing nuclei. They are only rarely observed and their significance is unknown.

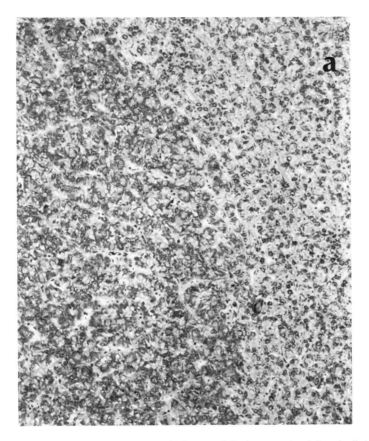

**FIG. 3a.** A large basophilic nodule from a fish that received 6 ppb dietary AFB₁ for 6 months. With the exception of basophilia, the nodular hepatocytes appear essentially normal and retain two-cell wide cords in most instances. Hematoxylin and eosin, × 320. (From Sinnhuber et al., ref. 85.)

The endpoint of the liver carcinogenic process in rainbow trout is the hepatocellular carcinoma frequently described by numerous authors. It consists of broad trabeculae of deeply basophilic cells, increased nuclear/cytoplasmic ratio, frequent mitoses, and it causes compression or invasion of surrounding normal tissue. It may consist of entirely trabecular elements (Fig. 3b and c), but more often it

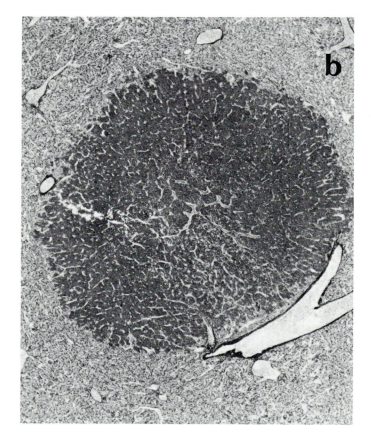

**FIG. 3b.**   A small trabecular hepatocellular carcinoma from a trout fed 800 ppm DMN for 12 months. Note the distinct basophilia, increased cord width, and beginning compression of surrounding normal tissue. Hematoxylin and eosin, × 80.

contains centrally located fibrous connective tissue and hyperplastic bile ducts (Fig. 3d). Bile ducts apparently are encompassed by tumor cells and stimulated to proliferate along with supportive connective tissue (35,85,112). Cholangiomas (Fig. 4a), or more rarely cholangiocarcinomas, also occur.

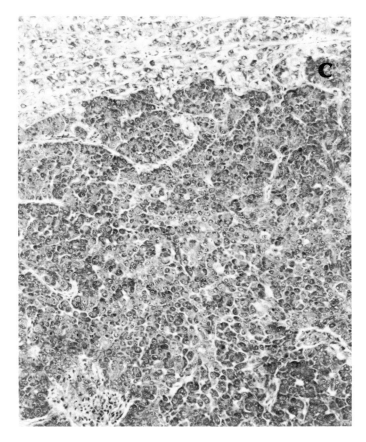

**FIG. 3c.** A portion of a large hepatocellular carcinoma from a trout fed 800 ppm DMN for 12 months. Cellular characteristics are similar to those of Figure 3b, but, in addition, frequent mitotic figures can be seen. Hematoxylin and eosin, × 320.

There have been attempts by several authors to distinguish between benign liver adenomas and malignant hepatocellular carcinomas on the basis of slight morphological differences (8,76). Generally these attempts have been unsuccessful since the criteria are arbitrary and not well defined. Scarpelli (76) sought to distinguish between putative adenomas and hepatomas by the biochemical

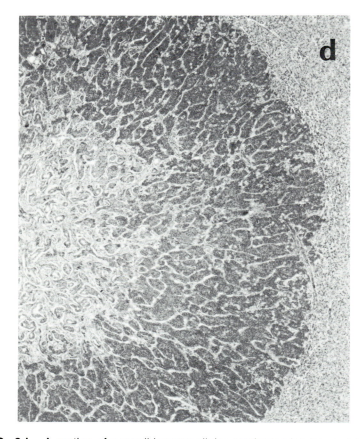

**FIG. 3d.** A portion of a small hepatocellular carcinoma having peripheral trabecular components and centrally located bile ducts supported by connective tissue. Tumor was initiated by 0.5 ppm sterigmatocystin embryo exposure. Hematoxylin and eosin, × 80. (From Hendricks et al. ref. 35.)

assay of several enzymes. Compared to normal liver tissue, there were increased activities of glutamic-pyruvic transaminase, glutamic oxaloacetic transaminase, lactic, malic, isocitric, and glucose-6-phosphate dehydrogenases, aldolase, leucyl aminopeptidase, both $Mg^{++}$- and $Ca^{++}$-activated adenosine triphosphatases, and decreased activities of succinic dehydrogenase, acid, alkaline, and

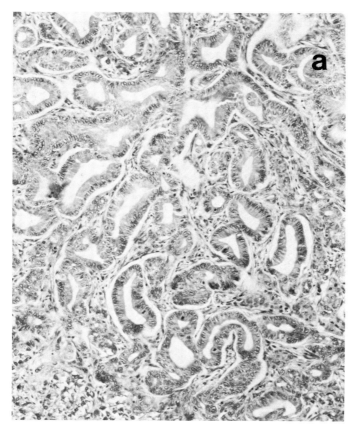

**FIG. 4a.** A portion of a cholangioma induced in rainbow trout liver by feeding 25 ppm, *p,p′*-DDT for 21 months. Note frequent mitotic figures in ductal epithelium and small portion of normal tissue at lower left. Hematoxylin and Eosin, × 80.

glucose-6-phosphatases in both adenomas and hepatomas; it was concluded that, enzymatically, adenomas and hepatomas were indistinguishable. The findings demonstrate that trout liver tumors are minimal deviation tumors, capable of performing the vital functions of the normal liver. It is not uncommon to observe normally swimming and feeding trout in which the normal liver has been almost totally replaced by single or multiple large tumor(s) (Fig. 4b).

At the FTNL, we have classified the grossly observable trout liver tumor as a hepatocellular carcinoma for the following reasons: (a) once induced, trout liver tumors continue to grow in the absence of the carcinogen, (b) metastases by cells of varying degrees of differentiation have been observed, so the diagnosis of malignancy on

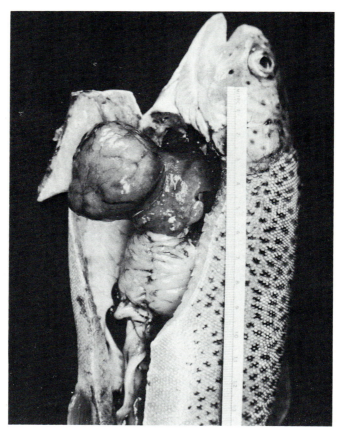

**FIG. 4b.** A yearling rainbow trout with a large hepatocellular carcinoma. Fish was fed GCK at 25% of the diet for 12 months. GCK contain CPFAs. (From Hendricks et al., ref. 33.)

the basis of the degree of anaplasia is unreliable (12,85,109), and (c) the potential for metastases is always present but usually not manifested until later in the trout's life, usually 3 to 6 years of age (6,7,8,85). Most of our experiments are terminated after 1 year, or, rarely, after 2 years, so we rarely observe any metastases. The fact that trout are poikilothermic and live at low environmental temperatures may partially explain why these tumors are so slow to metastasize. Trout liver tumors often cause the death of the fish before sufficient time has elapsed for metastases to occur. Sinnhuber et al. (87) reported heavy mortalities in mature (2-year-old) females with large liver tumors. Deaths were attributed to hemorrhaging from ruptured hepatic veins resulting from excessive weight of the large tumors.

In rats, all liver tumors are considered malignant since they all have the potential for malignant behavior (92,94). We feel the same is true for trout liver tumors, since the potential for malignant behavior always exists and often is manifested later in life. We also suggest the use of the term hepatocellular carcinoma rather than hepatoma, since the latter term is imprecise in its meaning with respect to malignancy.

*Metabolism*

Much evidence indicates that $AFB_1$ requires metabolic activation to exert its biologic effects (11,20–24,81,101–104). The ultimate carcinogenic form of $AFB_1$ appears to be the $AFB_1$-8.9-oxide (Fig. 1) (83,101–104). Much indirect evidence has shown that epoxidation at that site best explains the formation of a toxic, highly reactive, and mutagenic metabolite of $AFB_1$ by a cytochrome P-450-dependent microsomal oxidation, in which the 8,9-double bond is essential for the expression of these properties (20–23,81,101–104). Although the majority of these metabolic studies were conducted with rat liver preparations, Schoenhard et al. (81) showed that similar activation of $AFB_1$ to a toxic, reactive metabolite was performed by rainbow trout liver microsomes. Later, Stott and Sinnhuber (96) reported the mutagenicity of a metabolite formed by rainbow trout microsomes. The failure of $AFB_2$ (8,9-dihydro-$AFB_1$) to elicit a carcinogenic response in the extremely sensitive Shasta rainbow trout (9) further demonstrates the essential nature of the 8,9-double bond for carcinogenicity and points to the $AFB_1$-8,9-oxide as a probable ultimate carcinogen, even though the highly reactive metabolite cannot be isolated.

Alternate metabolic pathways result in the formation of other metabolites of $AFB_1$ that appear to be stages of detoxication and elimination from the body. Notable among these are the following: aflatoxicol (AFL), aflatoxin $M_1$ ($AFM_1$), aflatoxin $Q_1$ ($AFQ_1$), aflatoxin $P_1$ ($AFP_1$), aflatoxin $B_{2a}$ ($AFB_{2a}$), and aflatoxin $H_1$ ($AFH_1$) (Fig. 1).

*AFL.* AFL is the major *in vitro* metabolite produced by a soluble fraction enzyme of the trout liver (81). Campbell and Hayes (11) suggested that the enzyme responsible for the reduction of $AFB_1$ to AFL was NADPH-dependent 17-hydroxysteroid dehydrogenase, since it was completely inhibited by C-17 steroid hormones. Later *in vitro* studies have shown that AFL can be reconverted (dehydrogenated) to $AFB_1$ by postmitochondrial fractions of trout, rodent, and primate liver (57,74). Both reactions were uninhibited by carbon monoxide, indicating that they were not dependent on the cytochrome P-450 microsomal drug-metabolizing system (74).

The dietary exposure of rainbow trout to AFL has shown AFL to be a powerful carcinogen, about one-half as carcinogenic as $AFB_1$ at 8 months (82) (Table 11). Exposure of 14-day-old rainbow trout embryos to 0.5 ppm solutions of $AFB_1$ or AFL for 1 hr, however, resulted in similar tumor incidences at 12 months (53/100 for $AFB_1$ and 58/100 for AFL) (37). These results show that rainbow trout differ in sensitivity to AFL, depending on exposure route and possibly age. Relative mutagenicities of $AFB_1$ and AFL in the *Salmonella typhimurium* assay using a rat liver S-9 activating system were also quite different, and although AFL was the most mutagenic of all the $AFB_1$ metabolites, it was only about one-fourth as mutagenic as $AFB_1$ (119). Recent rat feeding trials with AFL have also shown AFL carcinogenic to rats but less so than $AFB_1$ (65).

Salhab and Edwards (74) showed a positive correlation between species sensitivity to $AFB_1$ and the ability of that animal to reduce

TABLE 11. Incidence of hepatocellular carcinoma in Shasta strain rainbow trout (S. gairdneri)[a]

| Toxicant in diet | 4-month sample (duplicate) carcinoma/40 trout | | % | 8-month sample (duplicate) carcinoma/40 trout | | % | 12-month sample (duplicate) carcinoma/sample | | % |
|---|---|---|---|---|---|---|---|---|---|
| None | 0 | 0 | 0 | 0 | 0 | 0 | 0/38 | 0/38 | 0 |
| 20 ppb $AFB_1$ | 0 | 0 | 0 | 18 | 27 | 56 | 29/37 | 33/38 | 83 |
| 29 ppb AFL | 0 | 0 | 0 | 11 | 10 | 26 | 25/31 | 21/26 | 81 |
| 61 ppb AFL' | 0 | 0 | 0 | 0 | 0 | 0 | 7/36 | 10/34 | 24 |
| 50 ppm CPFA | 0 | 0 | 0 | 1 | 1 | 3 | 16/38 | 13/36 | 39 |
| 20 ppb $AFB_1$ + 50 ppm CPFA | 6 | 3 | 11 | 39 | 38 | 96 | 32/32 | 32/32 | 100 |
| 29 ppb AFL + 50 ppm CPFA | 3 | 2 | 6 | 38 | 37 | 94 | 28/28 | 35/35 | 100 |
| 61 ppb AFL' + 50 ppm CPFA | 2 | 1 | 4 | 25 | 19 | 55 | 31/35 | 37/37 | 94 |

[a]Duplicate tanks of trout were fed a purified diet containing the toxicants AFL, $AFB_1$, and CPFA. Trout were randomly selected and sacrificed at 4-month intervals over a 12-month period. From Schoenhard et al. (82).

$AFB_1$ to AFL. It is still not known if AFL can be metabolized directly to the AFL-8,9-oxide or if it must be reconverted to $AFB_1$ to be activated. It appears highly possible, however, that the trout's metabolism of $AFB_1$ to AFL is an important factor in the extreme sensitivity of this species to $AFB_1$. The possibilities that the major detoxication metabolite (AFL) in rainbow trout can form a highly reactive epoxide or be reconverted to $AFB_1$ may help explain this sensitivity.

*$AFM_1$.* $AFM_1$ is the major *in vivo* metabolite formed by the bovine and is excreted into the milk after ingestion of $AFB_1$-contaminated feed (1). It is also formed *in vitro* by liver microsomal preparations from most animals, including rainbow trout, where it is a minor metabolite (56,57,81). The formation of $AFM_1$ from $AFB_1$ is a nonreversible, cytochrome P-450-mediated microsomal oxidation, and its conversion to a reactive metabolite, i.e., the epoxide, would be necessary for mutagenicity or carcinogenicity (11). The recent demonstration of $AFM_1$-DNA adducts in both rats and rainbow trout provide proof that $AFM_1$ can be metabolized to the 8,9-epoxide and covalently bind with DNA (R. Croy, *personal communication*).

Sinnhuber et al. (87) first demonstrated the carcinogenicity of $AFM_1$ in a whole animal system by producing hepatocellular carcinomas in rainbow trout (Table 12). Their results indicated that $AFM_1$ was about one-third as carcinogenic as $AFB_1$, a figure much higher than the relative mutagenicity of $AFB_1$ and $AFM_1$ in the *Salmonella* test (119). A high mortality was observed in females fed $AFM_1$ and held until 20 months. These fish were maturing sexually and had larger, more severe neoplastic lesions than similar aged males. Death resulted from hemorrhaging of hepatic veins, which may have resulted from weight stress on the veins or possible hormonal changes. Canton et al. (12) later confirmed Sinnhuber's results but did not assign a potency of $AFM_1$ relative to $AFB_1$. Wogan and Pagialunga (116) also found $AFM_1$ to be hepatocarcinogenic to rats. Recent results of $AFM_1$ exposure to rainbow trout embryos (37) (Table 10) showed that $AFM_1$ was only slightly carcinogenic, more nearly like the low mutagenicity shown by Wong and Hsieh (119). These results will require confirmation to decide what the true relative potency of $AFM_1$ and $AFB_1$ is and if it changes due to route of exposure.

$AFQ_1$. $AFQ_1$ is the major *in vitro* metabolite from monkey and human liver incubations of $AFB_1$ (10,46,59,60). It also is formed by a cytochrome P-450-mediated microsomal oxidation and would require activation to the 8,9-epoxide to be carcinogenic. In mutagenic studies, its relative potency was 83 times less than $AFB_1$ (119). Preliminary feeding trials of $AFQ_1$ with rainbow trout failed to produce a carcinogenic response at a level of 20 ppb (34). Embryo exposure to a 1.0 ppm solution also failed to elicit a carcinogenic response. Feeding trials with 100 ppb $AFQ_1$, however, did produce a significant incidence of liver tumors in rainbow trout, the only animal model in which the carcinogenicity of this compound has been shown (Table 13) (34). Its potency relative to $AFB_1$ was about 100 times less active, similar to Wong and Hsieh's (119) mutagenic data.

$AFB_{2a}$, $AFP_1$, *and* $AFH_1$. $AFB_{2a}$, a metabolite that lacks the terminal bifuran double bond, has not proved to be carcinogenic in rainbow trout by either dietary (J. D. Hendricks, *unpublished data*) or embryo exposure (37) (Table 10). It also showed no mutagenic activity in the *Salmonella* assay (119), indicating that its biologic activity is negligible.

$AFP_1$ is the major *in vivo* metabolite of $AFB_1$ produced by monkey and human liver (13,14). This o-demethylated form of $AFB_1$ had essentially no toxicity in the chick embryo test (95), or mutagenic activity in the *Salmonella* test (119), even though it retains the 8,9-double bond. Recent evidence has shown, however, that it binds to DNA in both rat and rainbow trout liver after *in vivo* exposure (R. Croy, *personal communication*), indicating that it probably forms a reactive 8,9-epoxide as do other $AFB_1$ metabolites. Two different exposures of rainbow trout embryos to $AFP_1$ (1 ppm for 24 hr and 5 ppm for 30 min) have been completed at our laboratory. Histo-

TABLE 12. Liver tumor incidence in rainbow trout fed $AFM_1$ and CPFA for 12 months[a]

| Diet no. | Diet description | 4 months | 8 months | 12 months | 16 months | Percent incidence at 16 months | Total volume of hepatoma tissue (mm³); 20 fish |
|---|---|---|---|---|---|---|---|
| 1 | Control diet (CD) | 0/40 | 0/20 | 1/40 | 0/20 | 0 | — |
| 2 | CD + 4 ppb $AFM_1$ | 2/40 | 0/20 | 6/46 | 8/20 | 40 | 1,662[b] |
| 3 | CD + 16 ppb $AFM_1$ | 0/40 | 0/20 | 30/43 | 13/20 | 65 | 9,706[c] |
| 4 | CD + 32 ppb $AFM_1$ | 2/40 | 3/20 | 28/46 | 19/20 | 95 | 24,254[d] |
| 5 | CD + 64 ppb $AFM_1$ | 0/40 | 1/20 | 30/50 | 19/20 | 95 | 86,753[e] |
| 6 | CD + 4 ppb $AFM_1$ + 100 ppm CPFA (S. foetida oil) | 6/40 | 14/20 | 42/63 | Terminated at 12 months | | |
| 7 | CD + 4 ppb $AFM_1$ + 100 ppm CPFA (H. syriacus oil) | 2/40 | 2/20 | 49/126 | Terminated at 12 months | | |
| 8 | CD + 4 ppb $AFB_1$ | 1/40 | 2/20 | 22/46 | 12/20 | 60 | 2,107 |
| 9 | CD + 4 ppb $AFB_1$ + 100 ppm CPFA (S. foetida oil) | 21/40 | 19/20 | Not sampled | 10/10 | 100 | — |

[a]Results expressed as number of trout with tumors/total number of trout.
[b]One large node not included (14,130 mm³).
[c]One large node not included (50,000 mm³).
[d]One large node not included (14,000 mm³).
[e]Two large nodes not included (20,300 and 8,000 mm³).
From Sinnhuber et al. (87).

TABLE 13. *Hepatocellular carcinoma incidences in rainbow trout fed experimental diets containing $AFQ_1$, $AFB_1$, and CPFA*

| Diet composition | Tank | Tumor incidence at[a] | | | | Combined 12 mo (%) | Average tumors/liver[b] | Average diameter of tumors (mm)[b] |
| | | 6 mo | 9 mo | 12 mo | | | | |
|---|---|---|---|---|---|---|---|---|
| Control | 1 | 0/10 | 0/10 | 0/60 | | 0/115 (0) | — | — |
| | 2 | 0/10 | 0/10 | 0/55 | | | | |
| Control + 100 ppb $AFQ_1$ | 1 | 0/10 | 0/10 | 4/59 | | 12/113 (11) | $1.1 \pm 0.3$ (12)[c] | $2.6 \pm 1.5$ (13)[d] |
| | 2 | 0/10 | 0/10 | 8/54 | | | | |
| Control + 50 ppm CPFA | 1 | 0/10 | 0/10 | 26/55 | | 44/107 (41) | $1.5 \pm 0.8$ (44)[c] | $5.5 \pm 5.9$ (64)[c] |
| | 2 | 0/10 | 1/10 | 18/52 | | | | |
| Control + 100 ppb $AFQ_1$ + 50 ppm CPFA | 1 | 3/10 | 3/10 | 56/60 | | 106/119 (89) | $3.8 \pm 3.7$ (106)[d] | $4.8 \pm 3.9$ (405)[c] |
| | 2 | 0/10 | 3/10 | 50/59 | | | | |
| Control + 4 ppb $AFB_1$ | 1 | 0/10 | 4/10 | 31/56 | | 55/114 (48) | $4.6 \pm 4.8$ (55)[d] | $2.6 \pm 2.2$ (253)[d] |
| | 2 | 0/10 | 1/10 | 24/59 | | | | |

[a]Results are expressed as number of trout with tumors/total number of trout.
[b]Results are given as means $\pm$ SD; numbers in parentheses indicate number of observations used in the calculation of mean and SD.
[c]Data significantly different at $p < 0.05$.
[d]Data significantly different at $p < 0.05$.
From Hendricks et al. (34).

pathologic examination of these trout livers is not complete, but gross observations revealed no tumors 12 months after exposure (J. D. Hendricks, *unpublished data*).

$AFH_1$, the reduced form of $AFQ_1$, was more mutagenic than $AFQ_1$ (119), but sufficient quantities of the compound have not been prepared to conduct a feeding or embryo exposure. When $AFH_1$ is available, the sensitive rainbow trout will be the animal of choice for testing, as it has been for many of the other $AFB_1$ metabolites.

*Sterigmatocystin and versicolorin A.* Wong et al. (120) identified versicolorin A (VA) and sterigmatocystin (ST) as precursors in the biosynthesis of $AFB_1$ by *Aspergillus flavus* and *A. parasiticus*. ST is also the end product of toxin biosynthesis by several other species of *Aspergillus* (38,71). Both compounds have an unsaturated bifuran structure in common with $AFB_1$, but they differ from $AFB_1$ in the remainder of the molecule (Fig. 1). Both compounds were mutagenic in the *Salmonella* assay, with VA about 1/20 and ST 1/10 as mutagenic as $AFB_1$ (120). The carcinogenicity of ST has been shown in several mammalian species by various exposure routes (19,68–70,106), and it is suspected of being one of the carcinogens contributing to human liver cancer in southern Africa (68,69). VA has not been tested for carcinogenicity in mammals. Rainbow trout embryos were exposed to aqueous solutions of both compounds (0.5 ppm ST) and (5 and 25 ppm VA) to test their carcinogenicity in trout. Tables 14 and 15 show the results of these exposures, verifying the carcinogenicity of ST and establishing for the first time the carcinogenicity of VA (35). Their relative carcinogenic potencies were also quite similar to the relative mutagenicities found by Wong et al. (120).

In all, the above mentioned dietary and embryo exposures of rainbow trout to the various mycotoxins, the carcinogenic response has been very consistent. Only hepatocellular carcinomas, rarely cholangiomas, were produced, and those produced by the various toxins were indistinguishable, indicating that the route of tumor initiation in the rainbow trout is similar throughout the mycotoxin group (Figs. 4c and d).

TABLE 14. *Hepatocellular carcinoma incidence resulting from exposure of 14-day rainbow trout embryos to ST and AFB,*

| Treatment | 12-mo tumor incidence[a] | Tumor diameter (mm)[b] |
|---|---|---|
| 0.5 ppm ST for 1 hr | 13/100 | 6.0 ± 5.9 (13) |
| 0.5 ppm AFB, for 1 hr | 53/100 | 4.9 ± 3.7 (87) |
| Water control for 1 hr | 0/100 | 0 ± 0 |

[a]Results expressed as number of tumor-bearing fish/total number of fish examined.
[b]Values are means ± SD. Numbers in parentheses are the total number of tumors.
From Hendricks et al. (35).

## Cyclopropenoid Fatty Acids

Following the discovery that aflatoxin was the principal causative agent of epizootic trout liver cancer, the next major related discovery concerned the role of cyclopropenoid fatty acids (CPFA) in trout liver cancer. Sinnhuber et al. (89,91) observed that naturally contaminated feedstuffs, such as cottonseed meals, produced a greater incidence and a more rapid growth rate of liver tumors than a control diet containing comparable levels of purified aflatoxin $B_1$. In subsequent experiments, Sinnhuber et al. (86) showed that dietary CPFAs, derived from *Sterculia foetida* oil and supplying 210 ppm sterculic and 10 ppm malvalic acids (Fig. 5) in triglyceride form, greatly increased the incidence and growth rate of trout liver cancer induced by dietary aflatoxin $B_1$ (Table 16). Previous work had shown that 220 ppm *Sterculia foetida* oil in the diet did not produce liver cancer in trout (89), so the effect of CPFA appeared to be a clear cut example of synergism or cocarcinogenesis (86). As shown in Table 16, gossypol, another naturally occurring polyphenolic compound in cottonseed, and 3-methylcoumarin, a compound with structural similarities to $AFB_1$, both increased the incidence of tumors at 12 and 15 months but not at 6 and 9 months as CPFA had done. Lee

TABLE 15. *Hepatocellular carcinoma incidence resulting from exposure of 21-day rainbow trout embryos to VA and $AFB_1$*

| Treatment | Preswimup mortalities[a] | No. of fish placed on feeding trial | Tumor incidence[b] 9 mo (%) | 12 mo (%) | Tumor diameter (mm)[c] |
|---|---|---|---|---|---|
| 5 ppm VA for 1 hr | 32 | 68[d] | — | 14/33 (42) | 2.9 ± 2.6 (25) |
| 25 ppm VA for 1 hr | 41 | 59 | — | 40/59 (68) | 3.8 ± 4.4 (54) |
| 0.5 ppm $AFB_1$ for 1 hr | 62 | 105 | 18/45 (40) | 41/60 (68) | 4.1 ± 4.5 (71) |
| 3% DMSO control for 1 hr | 52 | 105 | 0/44 (0) | 0/60 (0) | — |

[a]Number of fish.
[b]Results expressed as number of tumor-bearing fish/total number of fish examined; – indicates no sample was taken.
[c]Values are means ± SD. Numbers in parentheses are the total number of tumors.
[d]Due to asphyxiation, 35 additional fish in this group died early in the experiment.
From Hendricks et al. (35).

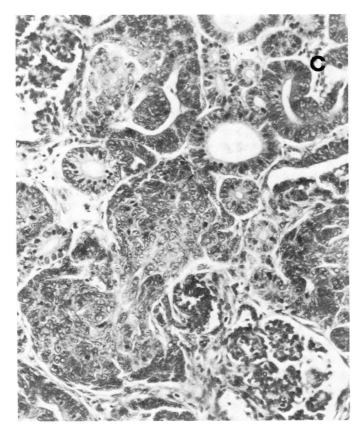

**FIG. 4c.** The advancing edge of a nephroblastoma initiated in a rainbow trout by embryo exposure to a 100 ppm solution of MNNG. Fish was killed at 12 months posttreatment. Note the basophilic neoplastic tissues *(center)* immediately adjacent to normal kidney tissue *(below and right)*, with no encapsulation. Hematoxylin and eosin, × 320. (From Hendricks et al., ref. 32.)

et al. (51 and 53) confirmed the synergistic effect of CPFA on $AFB_1$ carcinogenesis (Tables 2 and 3), both when it was fed concurrently with or after $AFB_1$ exposure. Lee et al. (51) also noted "spontaneous" tumors in the CPFA control diets, indicating that CPFAs may be carcinogenic themselves. Subsequent combined feedings of

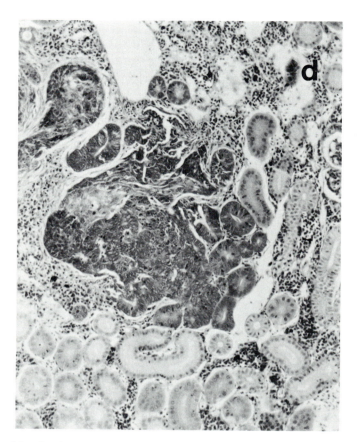

**FIG. 4d.** Portion of a nephroblastoma from a rainbow trout exposed to 100 ppm MNNG as an embryo and killed at 12 months. Note the abundant epithelial components (incompletely and imperfectly differentiated basophilic tubules and glomeruli) and sparse connective tissue stroma. Hematoxylin and eosin, × 512.

CPFA with various $AFB_1$ metabolites showed that the synergistic effect also occurred with $AFM_1$ (87), AFL (82), and $AFQ_1$ (34) (Tables 11, 12, and 13). The mechanism of CPFA synergistic activity on aflatoxin carcinogenesis remains obscure. Eisele et al. (17) and Loveland et al. (56) showed that CPFA depressed several MFO

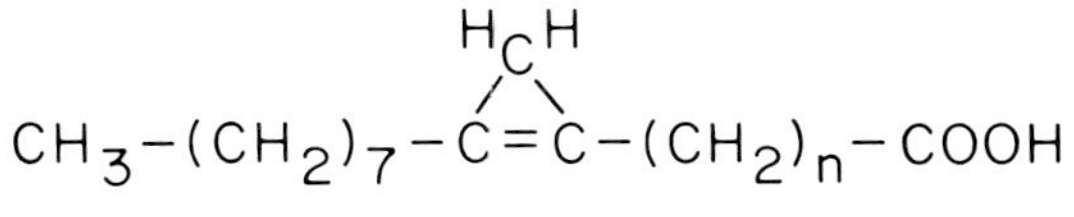

$$CH_3-(CH_2)_7-\underset{\overset{\diagup\diagdown}{\underset{C}{}}}{C}=C-(CH_2)_n-COOH$$

$$\overset{H_C H}{\diagup\diagdown}$$

n = 6  Malvalic acid

n = 7  Sterculic acid

**FIG. 5.**  Chemical structures of CPFAs.

enzyme activities in trout livers. Loveland et al. (56) also showed that CPFA significantly reduced *in vitro* AFL production from $AFB_1$ and completely inhibited $AFM_1$ formation. These studies show clearly that CPFAs affect the MFO system, but the changes produced are those that we would expect to result in lowered carcinogenicity rather than enhanced carcinogenicity. Previously cited studies have shown CPFA to be an effective synergist when fed together with $AFB_1$ (51,86,89) or subsequent to $AFB_1$ exposure (53), but we have not tested the effectiveness of preexposure to CPFA on $AFB_1$ carcinogenesis. At this time, it would appear that CPFAs act primarily as promotors of aflatoxin-initiated neoplasms, rather than affecting initiation, but the mechanism of promotion has not been investigated in detail.

Although early experiments (53,86,89) indicated that CPFAs were not carcinogenic, later combined CPFA and $AFB_1$ metabolite feeding experiments (34,51,82) clearly showed that the CPFA-control diets produced a significant incidence of hepatocellular carcinomas. This, again, may have resulted from dietary improvements that rendered the fish more susceptible to tumor development. A dose-response feeding trial with methyl sterculate substantiated these results and established the hepatocarcinogenicity of CPFA to rainbow trout (84). In that study, tumor incidence did not continue to increase with increasing dose level (Table 17). Maximum tumor incidence occurred at 45 ppm and decreased slightly at the two higher doses. This may be the result of the toxicity of high doses of CPFA causing an inhibitory effect on tumor growth. Finally, feeding trials with CPFA-containing natural cottonseed products, i.e., glandless (gossypol-free) cottonseed kernels (GCK) and cot-

TABLE 16. *Incidence of liver tumors in rainbow trout fed various test diets*

| Diet no. and description | Months | | | | |
|---|---|---|---|---|---|
| | 3 | 6 | 9 | 12 | 15 |
| 1) Control | 0/30 | 0/30 | 0/30 | 0/20 | 0/20 |
| 2) 4 ppb AFB$_1$ | 0/30 | 0/30 | 4/20 | 3/20 | 4/20 |
| 3) 8 ppb AFB$_1$ | 0/30 | 2/30 | 5/20 | 8/20 | 17/20 |
| 4) 20 ppb AFB$_1$ | 0/30 | 1/30 | 11/20 | 13/20 | 16/17 |
| 5) 4 ppb AFB$_1$ + 250 ppm gossypol | 0/30 | 0/30 | 5/20 | 6/20 | 12/20 |
| 6) 4 ppb AFB$_1$ + 50 ppb 3-methylcoumarin | 0/30 | 0/30 | 3/20 | 8/20 | 11/20 |
| 7) 1 ppm 3-methylcoumarin | 0/30 | 0/30 | 0/20 | 0/20 | 0/20 |
| 8) 4 ppb AFB$_1$ + 0.5% polymerized corn oil | 0/30 | 0/30 | 0/20 | 0/20 | 5/20 |
| 9) 4 ppb AFB$_1$ + 220 ppm CPFA | 0/30 | 27/30 | 20/20 | 9/10 | — |
| 10) 5% oxidized salmon oil | 0/30 | 0/30 | 0/20 | 0/20 | 0/20 |

From Sinnhuber et al. (86).

TABLE 17. *Hepatocellular carcinoma incidence in rainbow trout fed methyl sterculate for 11 months, the control diet for 7 additional months, and autopsied at 18 months*

| CPFA level (ppm) | 18-month liver tumor incidence |
|---|---|
| 0 | 0/37 |
| 5 | 1/40 |
| 15 | 13/40 |
| 45 | 15/38 |
| 135 | 11/39 |
| 405 | 10/38 |

From Sinnhuber et al. (84).

tonseed oil, have shown these products to be highly carcinogenic to rainbow trout (33) (Table 18) (Fig. 4b). The mechanism of tumor initiation is obscure, but the tumor produced is indistinguishable from those produced by the aflatoxins.

Sterculic acid has proved to be the most active of the two CPFAs (53). Recent experiments, however, with pure malvalic acid showed that it was both a synergist with $AFB_1$ and also carcinogenic by itself (J. D. Hendricks and J. E. Nixon, *unpublished data*), but only one-third or one-fourth as active as sterculic acid.

Doses of sterculic acid above 200 ppm in the diet are toxic to rainbow trout and cause severe necrosis of the liver (J. D. Hendricks, *unpublished observations*). Regeneration enables the livers to recover sufficiently to permit survival and growth, but succeeding generations of cells continue to be susceptible to chronic CPFA toxicity. Cells become enlarged, accumulate lipid and/or glycogen, develop bizarre, hyperchromatic nuclei, and develop unique fibrous-appearing striations in the cytoplasm (51,58,86,89,99). These striations consist of parallel arrays of endoplasmic reticulum at the ultrastructural level (80). Hepatocytes altered in these ways become degenerate and necrotic and are replaced by regenerated hepatocytes that appear to go through a similar cycle. Other generalized changes,

TABLE 18. *Liver cancer incidence in rainbow trout fed diets containing cottonseed products*

| Diet | After 6 months | After 9 months | After 12 months[a] | Percentage | Total number of tumors | Cumulative mortality |
|---|---|---|---|---|---|---|
| Control | | | | | | |
| Tank 1 | 0/10 | 0/10 | 0/26 | 0.0 | 0 | 4 |
| Tank 2 | 0/10 | 0/10 | 0/30 | 0.0 | 0 | 0 |
| Cottonseed oil | | | | | | |
| Tank 1 | 1/10 | 0/10 | 17/59 | 28.8 | 20 | 1 |
| Tank 2 | 0/10 | 0/10 | 21/58 | 36.2 | 27 | 2 |
| GCK | | | | | | |
| Tank 1 | 0/10 | 1/10 | 41/58 | 70.7 | 110 | 2 |
| Tank 2 | 0/10 | 3/10 | 46/58 | 75.9 | 106 | 2 |

[a]The number of controls sampled was smaller than the number of experimental animals because one-half of the controls also served as controls for another experiment that lasted an additional 3 months. Liver cancer was not detected in those controls at 15 months .
From Hendricks et al. (33).

including fibrosis, bile duct and vascular proliferation, disruption of normal hepatic architecture, and nodular hyperplasia of glycogen-laden hepatocytes (99) are prominent and appear to be irreversible.

Doses of sterculic acid below 100 ppm do not cause the initial necrosis described above, but the other chronic changes, namely, megalocytosis, lipid accumulation, cell striations, fibrosis, bile duct proliferation, and disruption of normal hepatic structure, are prominent.

The synergistic or carcinogenic properties of CPFA have not been unequivocally demonstrated in mammalian feeding trials (52,66), although Scarpelli (77,78) did demonstrate that CPFAs were mitogenic to rat liver and pancreas. The rabbit is the only mammal where liver pathology, similar to that seen in trout, has been observed (18).

## Nitrosamines and Nitrosamides

Ashley and Halver (8) first demonstrated the carcinogenicity of dimethylnitrosamine (DMN) to rainbow trout. They fed a series of doses ranging from 300 to 19,200 ppm in the diet for up to 20 months and produced high incidences of tumor-bearing fish—100% in the high dose group at 16 months. Grieco et al. (25) also fed DMN to rainbow trout, but at lower doses (3 to 800 ppm in the diet), for 12 months, and still achieved a high incidence of tumor-bearing animals at 12 and 18 months (Table 19). Comparison of these data with previously published rat data (107) showed that rainbow trout were of comparable sensitivity to DMN on a total dose level. The rat and trout dietary levels appear highly different, i.e., the high dose level for rats was 20 ppm and high dose for trout was 800 ppm. But because of the trout's highly efficient utilization of its food, the total amount of diet consumed is much less than for rats, so that on a total basis, the two dietary levels provide about the same total dose (Table 20).

Ashley (4) also reported the induction of several nephroblastomas in the trout fed DMN, but Grieco et al. (25) were unable to duplicate

TABLE 19. *Hepatocellular carcinoma in rainbow trout fed DMN[a]*

| DMN in diet (ppm) | Average total DMN dose (mg/trout) | Tumor incidence at 52-week sampling date (%)[b] | Tumor incidence at 78-week sampling date (%) |
|---|---|---|---|
| 0 | 0 | 0/60 (0) | 0/77 (0) |
| 3 | 0.72 | 0/60 (0) | 1/75 (1.3) |
| 200[c] | 47.8 | 2/60 (3.3) | 14/79 (17.7) |
| 200[c] | 45.6 | 4/60 (6.7) | 15/75 (20.0) |
| 400 | 96.4 | 20/60 (33.3) | 36/73 (49.3) |
| 800 | 195.9 | 44/60 (73.3) | 57/63 (90.5) |

[a]No tumors were observed at the 26-week sampling period.
[b]Number of trout with tumors/total number of trout.
[c]Half of these trout were fed DMN at 50 ppm for the first 12 weeks of the feeding experiment and were then inadvertently mixed with the remainder that had been fed DMN at 200 ppm for the first 12 weeks of the feeding experiment. Both groups of trout were fed DMN at 200 ppm for the duration of the feeding experiment.
From Grieco et al. (25).

these results. Perhaps the higher dose levels used by Ashley were responsible for the initiation of the nephroblastomas.

Initial trout embryo exposures to DMN were unsuccessful (37) even though high DMN concentrations (1 to 10,000 ppm in water) were used for 1-hr exposures. Since all previous embryo exposures had utilized mycotoxins, which are lipid-soluble compounds and only sparingly soluble in water, it was theorized that the water-soluble DMN was not moving from the water solution into the lipid-rich egg yolk. As a result, exposure time was increased to 24 hr, with aeration, for a 500 ppm solution of DMN, and a 17% incidence of liver tumors resulted at 1 year (37).

The results of only two exposures of rainbow trout to the direct acting nitrosamide, N-methyl-N'-nitro-N-nitrosoguanidine (MNNG), have been published. Oral exposure of this compound to rodents produces primarily stomach tumors (100). Gastric intubation of MNNG to rainbow trout resulted in the following tumor incidences: stomach adenomas (75%), liver hepatomas (81%), and kidney nephroblas-

TABLE 20. *Liver tumor incidence in rats fed DMN for 120 weeks*

| DMN in diet (ppm) | Average total DMN dose (mg/rat)[a] | Tumor incidence[b] (%) |
|---|---|---|
| 0 | 0 | 0/36 (0) |
| 2 | 25 | 1/26 (3.8) |
| 5 | 63 | 8/74 (10.8) |
| 10 | 126 | 2/5 (40.0) |
| 20 | 252 | 10/13 (76.9) |

[a]Calculations were based on a feed consumption of 15 g/day/rat for 7 days/week over a period of 120 weeks.
[b]Number of tumor-bearing rats/total number of rats. From Grieco et al. (25). Data tabulated from Terracini et al. (107).

tomas (17%) (45). Hendricks et al. (32) exposed rainbow trout embryos to 10, 30, and 100 ppm water solutions of MNNG for 1 hr and produced a high incidence of liver carcinomas and a low incidence of nephroblastomas (Fig. 4c and d), both in dose-dependent order (Table 21). In addition MNNG, at 100 ppm, had a peculiar sex reversal effect (female to male) on the trout. Thus, the embryo exposure model was also responsive to direct acting carcinogens, and, again, in dose-dependent fashion.

*Miscellaneous Chemical Carcinogens*

Halver (26) fed diets containing 13 different chemical carcinogens to rainbow trout fry for up to 20 months. The carcinogens were fed at five levels over a 256-fold range at $1/16$, $1/4$, 1, 4, and 16 times the dosage known to induce a high incidence of tumors in rodents. The following compounds were tested: urethane, carbon tetrachloride, carbarzone, thioacetamide, aminotriazole, 2-acetylaminofluorene, aminoazotoluene, dichloro-diphenyl-trichloroethane (DDT), *p*-dimethyl-aminoazobenzene, thiourea, dimethylnitrosamine, diethylstilbestrol, and tannic acid. Of these, only aminotriazole and thioacetamide failed to induce any liver tumors. Some of the other compounds, however, required feeding at very high doses to initiate tumor formation. Lee et al. (51) also fed 2-acetyl-aminofluorene to rainbow trout at 100 ppm but failed to produce tumors (Table 2).

At the FTNL, we have worked almost exclusively with aflatoxins and CPFAs until the present time. Presently, we are involved in testing a number of chemical carcinogens from different classes of compounds, several with extrahepatic organ specificity in rodents, to determine the versatility of rainbow trout as a broad-spectrum, carcinogenesis research animal. Most of these trials are presently underway and results are not available for this review.

We have confirmed the hepatocarcinogenicity of DDT for rainbow trout by feeding $p,p'$-DDT at 25 ppm for 21 months (J. D. Hendricks, *unpublished data*). Not only was there a significant response, tumor incidence was $31/59$ or 52% after 21 months continuous feeding, but there was a marked sexual response as well. Twenty-six out of 35 females (74%) had liver tumors, whereas only $5/24$ males (21%) had liver tumors. After 21 months on the DDT diet, these fish were sexually mature and ready to spawn, so the influence of female sex hormones may have contributed to the higher tumor incidence in females. Takashima (105) also has described the influence of female sex hormones on the spontaneous development of hepatic and cutaneous tumors in salmonids. His experiments provide convincing evidence that maturing females are more susceptible to tumor development and/or rapid tumor growth than are either immature females or mature or immature males. Sinnhuber et al. (87) also observed a sex-related mortality in tumor-bearing, sexually mature females, as mentioned previously. The mechanisms and specific hormones involved in this sex-related phenomenon deserve further study. The tumors were of two types: (a) typical hepatocellular carcinomas, as induced by aflatoxins and other trout carcinogens, and (b) cholangiomas/cholangiocarcinomas, which are only rarely seen with aflatoxins (J.D. Hendricks, *unpublished data*).

## Modifications of Carcinogenesis in Rainbow Trout

The aflatoxin-rainbow trout liver cancer model has been refined to the point that it serves as a convenient model system on which to study the effects of other modifiers on the carcinogenic process. The effects of CPFA as a probable promoter of aflatoxin carcinogenesis in trout has already been discussed. Other factors that have been studied at the FTNL include the effects of protein type and level on $AFB_1$ carcinogenesis, and the effects of MFO-inducing environmental contaminants [polychlorinated biphenyls, dieldrin, $p,p'$-dichloro-diphenyl-trichloroethylene (DDE)] on $AFB_1$ carcinogenesis.

### *Dietary Protein Effects*

Lee et al. (50) reported that both the level and type of dietary protein affected the carcinogenic response of rainbow trout to $AFB_1$. Low (32%) fish protein concentrate (FPC) in the diet appeared to repress tumor expression, while trout fed a high (49.5%) FPC diet had a higher tumor incidence than either the 32% FPC or the 32% or 49.5% casein diet fed fish. Subsequent unpublished results have confirmed the pronounced dietary protein effect on $AFB_1$ carcinogenesis. The mechanism again appears to be largely tumor promotion, since trout fed varying levels of FPC and casein do not show marked differences in liver MFO activity (97,98); also, trout exposed as embryos to $AFB_1$ and then fed the varying levels of FPC or casein show the same types of tumor incidence changes as when the protein diets were fed prior to and concurrently with the $AFB_1$ (J. D. Hendricks, *unpublished data*).

### *Effects of Liver MFO Inducers*

Since $AFB_1$ requires metabolic activation by the liver MFO system of animals, the potential for modifications of $AFB_1$ carcinogenesis by MFO-inducing environmental contaminants is high. We inves-

TABLE 21. *Tumor incidence in rainbow trout after embryonic exposure to MNNG*

| Treatment | 9-mo sample[a] | | 12-mo sample[a] | | No. of tumors/liver[b] | Tumor diameter (mm)[b] |
|---|---|---|---|---|---|---|
| | Nephro-blastomas (%) | Hepatocellular carcinomas (%) | Nephro-blastomas (%) | Hepatocellular carcinomas (%) | | |
| Sham control | 0/40 (0) | 0/40 (0) | 0/60 (0) | 0/60 (0) | 0 | 0 |
| 10 ppm MNNG | 0/40 (0) | 0/40 (0) | 1/60 (1.6) | 4/60 (6.7) | 1.5 ± 0.6 (4)[c] | 3.2 ± 3.4 (6) |
| 30 ppm MNNG | 1/40 (2.5) | 13/40 (32.5) | 3/60 (5.0) | 36/60 (60) | 2.1 ± 1.2 (36)[c] | 3.5 ± 3.7 (76) |
| 100 ppm MNNG | 3/40 (7.5) | 21/40 (52.5) | 5/60 (8.3) | 51/60 (85) | 3.4 ± 1.8 (51)[d] | 3.1 ± 2.4 (175) |

[a]Results expressed as number of tumor-bearing fish/total number of fish examined.
[b]Values are means ± SD. Numbers in parentheses are total number of observations.
[c,d]Values with different superscript letters were significantly different at $p < 0.001$.
From Hendricks et al. (32).

tigated this hypothesis by feeding rainbow trout 6 ppb $AFB_1$ together with 100 ppm Aroclor 1254 [a polychlorinated biphenyl (PCB) mixture known to induce the liver MFO system] along with appropriate positive and negative controls. As shown in Table 22, the combined feeding of $AFB_1$ and PCB dramatically reduced the incidence of tumors from the $AFB_1$ control (29). Several additional studies were then conducted to help determine the nature of this inhibition. First, to determine whether the inhibition occurred prior to or subsequent to tumor initiation, we exposed two groups of trout embryos to $AFB_1$ and then fed either control or 100 ppm PCB-containing diets to the resulting fry. As shown in Table 23, exposure to PCB after tumor initiation had little or no effect on tumor incidence (31). Secondly, we tested the effects of PCB exposure prior to $AFB_1$ challenge by feeding gravid female trout 200 ppm PCB in the diet for 2 months prior to spawning. Twenty-one-day embryos from a PCB-exposed female and a control female were each exposed to $AFB_1$ (0.5 ppm $AFB_1$ for 30 min) and fed the control diet from swimup for 12 months. Results of this experiment showed that prior exposure to PCB significantly increased the tumor incidence at both 9 and 12 months (Table 24) (36). MFO determinations on livers

TABLE 22. *Effect of dietary Aroclor 1254 (PCB) on aflatoxin-induced hepatocellular carcinoma incidence in rainbow trout*

| Diet | Tumor incidence 6 mo[a] | 9 mo | 12 mo | No. tumors/liver at 12 mo[b] | Tumor diameters at 12 mo (mm)[b] |
|---|---|---|---|---|---|
| CD | 0/10 | 0/10 | 0/68 | | |
| $AFB_1$ | 0/10[c] | 1/8 | 26/37 | 4.8 ± 5.1 (26) | 3.0 ± 2.7 (125) |
| PCB | 0/10 | 0/6 | 0/39 | | |
| $AFB_1$ + PCB | 0/10 | 1/10 | 14/46 | 2.4 ± 1.1 (14) | 2.1 ± 1.0 (33) |

[a]No tumors were seen in 1-, 2-, and 4-month samples. Results expressed as number of tumor-bearing fish/total number of fish.

[b]Mean ± SD. Number in parentheses indicates number of livers tested. Significantly different from other group by the use of Student's $t$-test ($p < 0.1$).

[c]Two small foci of basophilic cells were seen in histologic sections of these livers at 6 months.

From Hendricks et al. (29).

TABLE 23. *Growth, PCB content, and liver carcinoma incidence in rainbow trout 12 months after embryo exposure to AFB$_1$.[a,b]*

| Treatment[c] | Diet | Mortality | ppm PCB in whole fish[d] | Weight (g)[e] | Percent liver:body wt.[e,f] | Liver carcinoma incidence[g] | % | Tumor dia. (mm) | Tumors liver |
|---|---|---|---|---|---|---|---|---|---|
| Sham control | CD | 1 | 0.3 | 171.4 ± 40.3 (119) | 0.74 ± 0.11 (107) | 0/107 | 0 | — | — |
| 0.5 ppm AFB$_1$ (1 hr) | CD | 0 | — | 148.7 ± 35.0 (120)* | 0.72 ± 0.08 (41) | 79/120 | 65.8 | 4.6 ± 4.3 (132) 3 | 1.7 ± 0.9 (79) 1 |
| Sham control 0.5 ppm AFB$_1$ (1 hr) | CD + PCB | 0 | 75 | 143.7 ± 42.3 (120)* | 1.02 ± 0.16 (107)* | 1/108 | 0.9 | — | — |
| (1 hr) | CD + PCB | 0 | 76 | 154.6 ± 40.7 (120)* | 0.99 ± 0.18 (39)* | 69/108 | 63.9 | 5.5 ± 5.2 (121) | 1.8 ± 1.0 (69) |

[a]Trout were fed CD or CD + 100 ppm Aroclor 1254 (PCB) after embryo exposure.

[b]Body weight, percent liver:body wt., tumor diameter, and tumors/liver values are given as mean ± SD; the number of observations used in computation is given in parentheses.

[c]Sixty trout from each duplicate tank or 120 total trout (less mortalities) were included in each treatment group.

[d]Results obtained by analyzing 6 trout from each group or 12 total trout from each treatment group.

[e]Data with the superscript * were significantly different from the control at $p < 0.01$.

[f]Only livers without tumors were used to compute liver:body weight ratios.

[g]The number of fish is less due to the removal of 6 fish from each tank for PCB analysis. None were taken from the 0.5 ppm AFB, CD group. Results expressed as number of tumor bearing fish/total number of fish.

From Hendricks et al. (31).

TABLE 24. Incidence of hepatocellular carcinomas in rainbow trout exposed to $AFB_1$ as embryos

| Treatment group | 9 months | | | | 12 months | | | |
| --- | --- | --- | --- | --- | --- | --- | --- | --- |
| | Incidence[a] | % | Tumors/liver[b] | Av. dia. (mm)[b] | Incidence[a] | % | Tumors/liver[b] | Av. dia. (mm)[b] |
| OMP-female-control | 0/41 | 0 | 0 | 0 | 0/58 | 0 | 0 | 0 |
| OMP-female-$AFB_1$ | 15/40 | 37.5 | 1.3 ± 0.6 (15) | 2.5 ± 1.5 (19) | 39/59 | 66 | 1.8 ± 0.8 (39) | 4.5 ± 4.7 (70) |
| PCB-female-control | 0/40 | 0 | 0 | 0 | 0/56 | 0 | 0 | 0 |
| PCB-female-$AFB_1$ | 24/40 | 60[c] | 1.8 ± 1.0 (24) | 3.8 ± 3.2 (43) | 53/57 | 93[d] | 2.3 ± 1.6 (53) | 5.2 ± 4.5 (120) |

[a]Results expressed as number of tumor-bearing fish/total number of fish.
[b]Values are given as mean ± SD; total number of observations in parentheses.
[c]Significantly higher at $p < 0.025$.
[d]Significantly higher at $p < 0.001$.
From Hendricks et al. (36).

removed from 1-week-old sac fry from each group showed that enzyme activity was present in these very young individuals and also was inducible by PCB. We have also shown that the dietary level of PCB used in these experiments (100 ppm) does significantly induce selected MFO parameters of the trout liver (108). Additional studies on these interactions are in progress, but these results indicate several possible mechanisms of action. First, prior exposure of trout to PCB results in MFO induction, increased $AFB_1$ metabolism to the 8,9-epoxide, and enhanced carcinogenesis. Second, PCBs have no apparent promoting or inhibiting effect on previously initiated tumors in rainbow trout. Third, concurrent feeding of $AFB_1$ and PCB resulted in reduced $AFB_1$ metabolism to the epoxide, due to competitive inhibition for MFO components since PCBs are metabolized by the same system and were present in great excess compared to $AFB_1$. Similar competitive inhibition has been described for other combined carcinogen-inducer exposures (72). Although high doses of PCB have caused hepatic tumors in rodents (44), our 1-year exposures to low levels of PCB (100 ppm or less) (29,31,55) have caused no tumors in rainbow trout. Higher dose levels are currently under test.

Combined feeding of $AFB_1$ (6 ppb) and dieldrin (5 ppm) produced a slight but nonsignificant increase in tumor incidence over the $AFB_1$ control (30), but combined feeding of $AFB_1$ (6 ppb)and $p,p'$-DDE (5 ppm) had no effect on tumor incidence (J. D. Hendricks, *unpublished data*).

This review of the "state of the art" with regard to experimental carcinogenesis in salmonids suggests several conclusions. First, rainbow trout have served an important role in elucidating the metabolism and carcinogenicity of $AFB_1$ and its metabolites due to their high sensitivity to mycotoxins. Second, experience has shown that rainbow trout can be reared more economically than rodents, so there is a rational basis for their use in selected studies. Third, comparison of their metabolic characteristics indicate many similarities with mammals, and differences that do exist are often no greater than interspecific differences between "accepted" mammalian species. Fourth, rainbow trout, or fish in general, obviously can never totally replace mammals as experimental animals for biomedical research, since some vital systems, i.e., respiration, are radically different, both anatomically and functionally. However, there does appear to be a need for aquatic species in an increasing number of specific, particularly environmentally related, areas of biomedical research, and the rainbow trout has proved to be especially adaptable to many of these needs.

## CHEMICAL CARCINOGENESIS IN AQUARIUM FISHES

The use of sensitive, small aquarium fishes for carcinogenic research presents several advantages over larger fish like the salmonids. These include: (a) fish-holding facility requirements are minimal, (b) water temperature and quantity are less critical, (c) total research costs are much less, and (d) shorter life span accelerates tumor development. On the negative side, however, is the fact that their small size precludes or complicates *in vitro* metabolic studies where sizable quantities of liver are required, and it is very difficult to determine exact dosage received by aquarium fish with either dietary or water exposure.

Induction of tumors by chemical carcinogens in small aquarium fish has been reported by several investigators (2,3,39,41–43,54, 61,67,75,93) and recently reviewed by Matsushima and Sugimura (62). These studies have dealt with several classes of chemical carcinogens, including: (a) polycyclic aromatic hydrocarbons 7,12-dimethylbenz[a]anthracene (DMBA) and 3-methylcholanthrene (MCA), which were noncarcinogenic to guppies, *Lebistes reticulatus*, (67); (b) aromatic amines N-2-fluorenylacetamide (2-FAA), which was hepatocarcinogenic to guppies by dietary exposure (67,75); (c) azo compounds 4-dimethyl-aminoazobenzene (DAB) and *o*-aminoazotoluene (AAT), hepatocarcinogenic to guppies by dietary exposure (42,67); (d) nitroso compounds (DENA), hepatocarcinogenic by water exposure to zebra danio (*Brachydanio rerio*) (93), guppies (41,43,67), and medakas (*Oryzios latipes*) (39); (DMN), hepatocarcinogenic to guppies by water exposure (41,43,67) and by dietary exposure (61,75); nitrosomorpholine (NM), hepatocarcinogenic to guppies by water exposure (67); and (e) mycotoxins AFB$_1$, carcinogenic by dietary exposure to the liver of guppies (61,75) and ST, carcinogenic to the liver of guppies by dietary exposure (61).

More recent experimentation with aquarium fish carcinogenesis has focused on the medaka (*Oryzias latipes*) as the apparent species of choice (2,3,40,47–49). Aoki and Matsudaira (2,3) reported the hepatocarcinogenicity of another compound, methylazoxymethanol acetate, to the medaka by water exposure. Stanton (93) earlier had demonstrated the carcinogenicity of cycad nut meal by feeding of methylazoxymethanol β-D-glucoside in the water to the zebra danio *Brachydanio rerio* and the guppy. Methylazoxymethanol is the active compound in the *Cycas circinalis* plant.

The studies by Kyono and Egami (48), Kyono (47), Ishikawa and Takayama (40), and Kyono et al. (49) focus on defining specific aspects of the medaka-DENA water exposure model system, much in the same way that the rainbow trout-AFB$_1$ model system has been developed. Thus, Kyono and Egami (48) and Kyono (47) investigated the effects of temperature during and after DENA exposure and found marked increases in carcinogenicity with elevated temperatures. Low temperatures at exposure time inhibited tumor formation. Ishikawa and Takayama (40) investigated the pathogenesis of tumor development and the effects of length of exposure time on tumor development. At a dose of 45 ppm dissolved in the water, no tumors developed after 3-day or 1-week exposures, but increasing incidences resulted from 2-, 4-, and 6-week exposures. Although it is difficult to compare the effective dose given (concentration × time), it would appear from rainbow trout embryo exposures to DENA and DMN that the trout is more sensitive than the medaka, since the exposure time required is only 24 hr, but the dose used is considerably higher (500 to 1,000 ppm). Finally, Kyono et al. (49) studied DNA labeling and DNA content during DENA-induced liver carcinogenesis in the medaka.

Although the level of effort in aquarium fish chemical carcinogenesis has been much less than that for salmonid chemical carcinogenesis, interest in aquarium fish appears high and the future will probably reveal a much greater effort in this area. As with salmonids, carcinogenesis research with aquarium fishes has involved primarily liver carcinogens. Although liver carcinogenesis is a convenient and logical starting place in developing model systems for cancer research, it often results in the conclusion, by critics of aquatic models, that fish respond only to liver carcinogens and that there are already adequate model systems available in this area. Thus, there is a need for a concerted effort to determine the response of aquarium fish to other organ-specific carcinogens. Only in this way can their desirability as model systems for other types of cancer research or as general test species be evaluated.

## ACKNOWLEDGMENTS

This work was supported by U.S. Public Health Service Grants ES 00210, ES 01926, and ES 00541 from the National Institute of Environmental Health Sciences. Technical paper No. 5780 of the Oregon Agricultural Experiment Station, Oregon State University.

## REFERENCES

1. Allcroft, R., and Carnaghan, R. B. A. (1963): Groundnut toxicity: An examination for toxin in human food products from animals fed toxic groundnut meal. *Vet. Rec.*, 75:259–263.
2. Aoki, K., and Matsudaira, H. (1977): Induction of hepatic tumors in a teleost (*Oryzias latipes*) after treatment with methylazoxymethanol acetate: Brief communication. *J. Natl. Cancer Inst.*, 59:1,747–1,749.
3. Aoki, K., and Matsudaira, H. (1980): Induction of hepatic tumors after treatment with MAM acetate in *Oryzias latipes* and its inhibition by previous irradiation with X-rays. In: *Radiation Effects on Aquatic Organisms*, edited by N. Egami, pp. 209–211. Japan Sci. Soc. Press, Tokyo/Univ. Park Press, Baltimore.
4. Ashley, L. M. (1969): Experimental fish neoplasia. In: *Fish in Research*, edited by O. W. Neuhaus and J. E. Halver, pp. 23–43. Academic Press, New York.
5. Ashley, L. M. (1970): Pathology of fish fed aflatoxins and other antimetabolites. In: *A Symposium on Diseases of Fishes and Shellfishes*, vol. 5, edited by S. F. Snieszko, pp. 366–379. American Fisheries Society, Washington, D. C.
6. Ashley, L. M. (1973): Animal model: Liver cell carcinoma in rainbow trout. *Am. J. Pathol.*, 72:345–348.

7. Ashley, L. M., and Halver, J. E. (1963): Multiple metastasis of rainbow trout hepatoma. *Trans. Am. Fish Soc.*, 92:365–371.
8. Ashley, L. M., and Halver, J. E. (1968): Dimethylnitrosamine-induced hepatic cell carcinoma in rainbow trout. *J. Natl. Cancer Inst.*, 41:531–552.
9. Ayres, J. L., Lee, D. J., Wales, J. H., and Sinnhuber, R. O. (1971): Aflatoxin structure and hepatocarcinogenicity in rainbow trout (*Salmo gairdneri*). *J. Natl. Cancer Inst.*, 46:561–564.
10. Buchi, G. H., Muller, P. M., Roebuck, B. D., and Wogan, G. N. (1974): Aflatoxin $Q_1$: A major metabolite of aflatoxin $B_1$ produced by human liver. *Res. Commun. Chem. Pathol. Pharmacol.*, 8:585–592.
11. Campbell, T. C., and Hayes, J. R. (1976): The role of aflatoxin metabolism in its toxic lesion. *Toxicol. Appl. Pharmacol.*, 35:199–222.
12. Canton, J. H., Kroes, R., van Logten, M. J., van Schothorst, M., Stavenuiter, J. F. C., and Verhulsdonk, C. A. H. (1975): The carcinogenicity of aflatoxin $M_1$ in rainbow trout. *Food Cosmet. Toxicol.*, 13:441–443.
13. Dalezios, J. I., Hsieh, D. P. H., and Wogan, G. N. (1973): Excretion and metabolism of orally administered aflatoxin $B_1$ by rhesus monkeys. *Food Cosmet. Toxicol.*, 11:605–616.
14. Dalezios, J. I., Wogan, G. N., and Weinreb, S. M. (1971): Aflatoxin $P_1$: A new aflatoxin metabolite in monkeys. *Science*, 171:584–585.
15. Dawe, C. (1969): Phylogeny and oncogeny. *Natl. Cancer Inst. Monogr.*, 31:1–39.
16. Dawe, C. J., and Harshbarger, J. C. (1975): Neoplasms in feral fishes: Their significance to cancer research. In: *The Pathology of Fishes*, edited by W. E. Ribelin and G. Migaki, pp. 871–894. University of Wisconsin Press, Madison.
17. Eisele, T. A., Nixon, J. E., Pawlowski, N. E., and Sinnhuber, R. O. (1978): Effects of dietary cyclopropene fatty acids on the mixed-function oxidase system of the rainbow trout. *J. Environ. Pathol. Toxicol.*, 1:773–778.
18. Ferguson, T. L., Wales, J. H., Sinnhuber, R. O., and Lee, D. J. (1976): Cholesterol levels, atherosclerosis, and liver morphology in rabbits fed cyclopropenoid fatty acids. *Food Cosmet. Toxicol.*, 14:15–18.
19. Fujii, K., Kurata, H., Odashima, S., and Hatsuda, Y. (1976): Tumor induction by a single subcutaneous injection of sterigmatocystin in newborn mice. *Cancer Res.*, 36:1,615–1,618.
20. Garner, R. C. (1973): Chemical evidence for the formation of a reactive aflatoxin $B_1$ metabolite by hamster liver microsomes. *Fed. Eur. Biochem. Soc. Letters*, 36:261–264.
21. Garner, R. C., Miller, E. C., and Miller, J. A. (1972): Liver microsomal metabolism of aflatoxin $B_1$ to a reactive derivative toxic to *Salmonella typhimurium* TA 1530. *Cancer Res.*, 32:2,058–2,066.
22. Garner, R. C., Miller, E. C., Miller, J. A., Garner, J. V., and Hanson, R. S. (1971): Formation of a factor lethal for *S. typhimurium* TA 1530 and TA 1531 on incubation of aflatoxin $B_1$ with rat liver microsomes. *Biochem. Biophys. Res. Commun.*, 45:774–780.

23. Garner, R. C., and Wright, C. M. (1973): Induction of mutations in DNA-repair deficient bacteria by a liver microsomal metabolite of aflatoxin $B_1$. *Br. J. Cancer*, 28:544–551.

24. Garner, R. C., and Wright, C. M. (1975): Binding of [$^{14}$C]aflatoxin $B_1$ to cellular macromolecules in the rat and hamster. *Chem. Biol. Interact.*, 11:123–131.

25. Grieco, M. P., Hendricks, J. D., Scanlan, R. A., and Sinnhuber, R. O. (1978): Carcinogenicity and acute toxicity of dimethylnitrosamine in rainbow trout (*Salmo gairdneri*). *J. Natl. Cancer Inst.*, 60:1,127–1,131.

26. Halver, J. E. (1967): Crystalline aflatoxin and other vectors for trout hepatoma. In: *Trout Hepatoma Research Conference Papers*, edited by J. E. Halver and I. A. Mitchell, Res. Rept. 70:78–102. Bureau of Sport Fisheries and Wildlife, Washington, D. C.

27. Halver, J. E. (1969): Aflatoxicosis and trout hepatoma. In: *Aflatoxins*, edited by L. A. Goldblatt, pp. 265–306. Academic Press, New York.

28. Halver, J. E., and Mitchell, I. A., editors (1967): *Trout Hepatoma Research Conference Papers*. Bureau of Sport Fisheries and Wildlife, Washington, D. C.

29. Hendricks, J. D., Putnam, T. P., Bills, D. D., and Sinnhuber, R. O. (1977): Inhibitory effect of a polychlorinated biphenyl (Aroclor 1254) on aflatoxin $B_1$ carcinogenesis in rainbow trout (*Salmo gairdneri*). *J. Natl. Cancer Inst.*, 59:1,545–1,551.

30. Hendricks, J. D., Putnam, T. P., and Sinnhuber, R. O. (1979): Effect of dietary dieldrin on aflatoxin $B_1$ carcinogenesis in rainbow trout (*Salmo gairdneri*). *J. Environ. Pathol. Toxicol.*, 2:719–728.

31. Hendricks, J. D., Putnam, T. P., and Sinnhuber, R. O. (1980): Null effect of dietary Aroclor 1254 on hepatocellular carcinoma incidence in rainbow trout (*Salmo gairdneri*) exposed to aflatoxin $B_1$ as embryos. *J. Environ. Pathol. Toxicol.*, 4:9–16.

32. Hendricks, J. D., Scanlan, R. A., Williams, J. L., Sinnhuber, R. O., and Grieco, M. P. (1980): Carcinogenicity of N-methyl-N'-nitro-N-nitrosoguanidine to rainbow trout (*Salmo gairdneri*) exposed as embryos. *J. Natl. Cancer Inst.*, 64:1,511–1,519.

33. Hendricks, J. D., Sinnhuber, R. O., Loveland, P. M., Pawlowski, N. E., and Nixon, J. E. (1980): Hepatocarcinogenicity of glandless cottonseeds and cottonseed oil to rainbow trout (*Salmo gairdneri*). *Science*, 208:309–311.

34. Hendricks, J. D., Sinnhuber, R. O., Nixon, J. E., Wales, J. H., Masri, M. S., and Hsieh, D. P. H. (1980): Carcinogenic response of rainbow trout (*Salmo gairdneri*) to aflatoxin $Q_1$ and synergistic effect of cyclopropenoid fatty acids. *J. Natl. Cancer Inst.*, 64:523–527.

35. Hendricks, J. D., Sinnhuber, R. O., Wales, J. H., Stack, M. E., and Hsieh, D. P. H. (1980): Hepatocarcinogenicity of sterigmatocystin and versicolorin A to rainbow trout (*Salmo gairdneri*) embryos. *J. Natl. Cancer Inst.*, 64:1,503–1,509.

36. Hendricks, J. D., Stott, W. T., Putnam, T. P., and Sinnhuber, R. O. (1980): Enhancement of aflatoxin $B_1$ hepatocarcinogenesis in rainbow trout *(Salmo*

*gairdneri*) embryos by prior exposure of gravid females to dietary Aroclor 1254. In: *Aquatic Toxicology and Hazard Assessment: Fourth Conference.* ASTM STP 737, edited by D. R. Branson and K. L. Dickson, pp. 203–214, American Society for Testing and Materials.

37. Hendricks, J. D., Wales, J. H., Sinnhuber, R. O., Nixon, J. E., Loveland, P. M., and Scanlan, R. A. (1980): Rainbow trout (*Salmo gairdneri*) embryos: A sensitive animal model for experimental carcinogenesis. *Fed. Proc.,* 39:3,222–3,229.

38. Hsieh, D. P. H., Singh, R., Yao, R. C., and Bennett, J. W., (1978): Anthraquinones in the biosynthesis of sterigmatocystin by *Aspergillus versicolor. Appl. Environ. Microbiol.,* 35:980–982.

39. Ishikawa, T., Shimamine, T., and Takayama, S. (1975): Histologic and electron microscopy observations on diethylnitrosamine-induced hepatomas in small aquarium fish (*Oryzias latipes*). *J. Natl. Cancer Inst.,* 55:906–916.

40. Ishikawa, T., and Takayama, S. (1979): Importance of hepatic neoplasms in lower vertebrate animals as a tool in cancer research. *J. Toxicol. Environ. Health,* 5:537–550.

41. Khudoley, V. V. (1971): The induction of hepatic tumors by nitrosamines in aquarium fish (*Lebistes reticulatus*). *Uop. Onkol.,* 17:67–72.

42. Khudoley, V. V. (1972): Induction of liver tumors by some azo compounds in aquarium guppies [*Lebistes reticulatus* (Peters)]. *J. Ichthyol.,* 12:319–324.

43. Khudoley, V. V. (1973): Morphological changes in the liver of fish (*Lebistes reticulatus*) under the action of diethyl- and dimethyl-nitrosamines. *Uop. Onkol.,* 19:88–94.

44. Kimbrough, R. D., and Linder, R. E. (1974): Induction of adenofibrosis and hepatomas of the liver in BALB/cJ mice by polychlorinated biphenyls (Aroclor 1254). *J. Natl. Cancer Inst.,* 53:547–552.

45. Kimura, I., Miyaki, T., and Yoshizaki, K. (1976): Induction of tumors of the stomach, of the liver, and of the kidney in rainbow trout by intrastomach administration of N-methyl-N-nitroso-N'-nitrosoguanidine (MNNG). *Proc. Jap. Cancer Assoc.,* 35:16.

46. Krieger, R. I., Salhab, A. S., Dalezios, J. I., and Hsieh, D. P. H. (1975): Aflatoxin $B_1$ hydroxylation by hepatic microsomal preparations from the rhesus monkey. *Food Cosmet. Toxicol.,* 13:211–219.

47. Kyono, Y. (1978): Temperature effects during and after the diethylnitrosamine treatment on liver tumorigenesis in the fish *Oryzias latipes. Europ. J. Cancer,* 14:1,089–1,097.

48. Kyono, Y., and Egami, N. (1977): The effect of temperature during the diethylnitrosamine treatment on liver tumorigenesis in the fish *Oryzias latipes. Eur. J. Cancer,* 13:1,191–1,194.

49. Kyono, Y., Shima, A., and Egami, N. (1979): Changes in the labeling index and DNA content of liver cells during diethylnitrosamine-induced liver tumorigenesis in *Oryzias latipes. J. Natl. Cancer Inst.,* 63:71–74.

50. Lee, D. J., Sinnhuber, R. O., Wales, J. H., and Putnam, G. B. (1977): Effect of dietary protein on the response of rainbow trout (*Salmo gairdneri*) to aflatoxin $B_1$. *J. Natl. Cancer Inst.*, 60:317–320.

51. Lee, D. J., Wales, J. H., Ayres, J. L., and Sinnhuber, R. O. (1968): Synergism between cyclopropenoid fatty acids and chemical carcinogens in rainbow trout (*Salmo gairdneri*). *Cancer Res.*, 28:2,312–2,318.

52. Lee, D. J., Wales, J. H., and Sinnhuber, R. O. (1969): Hepatoma and renal tubule adenoma in rats fed aflatoxin and cyclopropenoid fatty acids. *J. Natl. Cancer Inst.*, 43:1,037–1,044.

53. Lee, D. J., Wales, J. H., and Sinnhuber, R. O. (1971): Promotion of aflatoxin-induced hepatoma growth in trout by methyl malvalate and sterculate. *Cancer Res.*, 31:960–963.

54. Levy, B. M. (1962): Experimental induction of tumor-like lesions of the notochord of fish. *Cancer Res.*, 22:441–444.

55. Lieb, A. J., Bills, D. D., and Sinnhuber, R. O. (1974): Accumulation of dietary polychlorinated biphenyls (Aroclor 1254) by rainbow trout (*Salmo gairdneri*). *J. Agric. Food Chem.*, 22:638–642.

56. Loveland, P. M., Nixon, J. E., Pawlowski, N. E., Eisele, T. A., Libbey, L. M., and Sinnhuber, R. O. (1979): Aflatoxin $B_1$ and aflatoxicol metabolism in rainbow trout (*Salmo gairdneri*) and the effects of dietary cyclopropene. *J. Environ. Pathol. Toxicol.*, 2:707–718.

57. Loveland, P. M., Sinnhuber, R. O., Berggren, K. E., Libbey, L. M., Nixon, J. E., and Pawlowski, N. E. (1977): Formation of aflatoxin $B_1$ from aflatoxicol by rainbow trout (*Salmo gairdneri*) liver *in vitro*. *Res. Commun. Chem. Pathol. Pharmacol.*, 16:167–170.

58. Malevski, Y., Wales, J. H., and Montgomery, M. W. (1974): Liver damage in rainbow trout (*Salmo gairdneri*) fed cyclopropenoid fatty acids. *J. Fish Res. Board Can.*, 31:1,397–1,400.

59. Masri, M. S., Booth, A. N., and Hsieh, D. P. H. (1974): Comparative metabolic conversion of aflatoxin $B_1$ to $M_1$ and $Q_1$ by monkey, rat, and chicken liver. *Life Sci.*, 15:203–212.

60. Masri, M. S., Haddon, W. F., Lundin, R. E., and Hsieh, D. P. H. (1974): Aflatoxin $Q_1$, a newly identified major metabolite of aflatoxin $B_1$ in monkey liver. *J. Agric. Food Chem.*, 22:512–515.

61. Matsushima, T., Sato, S., Hara, K., Sugimura, T., and Takashima, F. (1975): Bioassay of environmental carcinogens with the guppy *Lebistes reticulatus*. *Mutat. Res.*, 31:265.

62. Matsushima, T., and Sugimura, T. (1976): Experimental carcinogenesis in small aquarium fishes. *Prog. Exp. Tumor Res.*, 20:367–379.

63. Mawdesley-Thomas, L. E. (1972): Some tumours of fish. In: *Diseases of Fish*, edited by L. E. Mawdesley-Thomas, *Symp. Zool. Soc. Lond.*, 30:191–284. Academic Press, New York.

64. Mawdesley-Thomas, L. E. (1975): Neoplasia in fish. In: *The Pathology of Fishes*, edited by W. E. Ribelin and G. Migaki, pp. 805–870. University of Wisconsin Press, Madison.

65. Nixon, J. E., Hendricks, J. D., Pawlowski, N. E., Loveland, P. M., and Sinnhuber, R. O. (1981): Carcinogenicity of aflatoxicol in Fischer rats. *J. Natl. Cancer Inst.*, 66:1,159–1,163.
66. Nixon, J. E., Sinnhuber, R. O., Lee, D. J., Landers, M. K., and Harr, J. R. (1974): Effect of cyclopropenoid compounds on the carcinogenic activity of diethylnitrosamine and aflatoxin B$_1$ in rats. *J. Natl. Cancer Inst.*, 53:453–458.
67. Pliss, G. B., and Khudoley, V. V. (1975): Tumor induction by carcinogenic agents in aquarium fish. *J. Natl. Cancer Inst.*, 55:129–136.
68. Purchase, I. F., and van der Watt, J. J. (1968): Carcinogenicity of sterigmatocystin. *Food Cosmet. Toxicol.*, 6:555–556.
69. Purchase, I. F., and van der Watt, J. J. (1970): Carcinogenicity of sterigmatocystin. *Food Cosmet. Toxicol.*, 8:289–295.
70. Purchase, I. F., and van der Watt, J. J. (1973): Carcinogenicity of sterigmatocystin to rat skin. *Toxicol. Appl. Pharmacol.*, 26:274–281.
71. Rabie, C. J., Steyn, M., and van Schalkwyk, G. C. (1977): New species of *Aspergillus* producing sterigmatocystin. *Appl. Environ. Microbiol.*, 33:1,023–1,025.
72. Razzouk, C., Agazzi-Leonard, E., Batardy-Gregoire, M., Mercier, M., Poncelet, F., and Roberfroid, M. (1980): Competitive inhibitory effect of microsomal N-hydroxylase, a possible explanation for the *in vivo* inhibition of 2-acetylaminofluorene carcinogenicity by 3-methylcholanthrene. *Toxicol. Lett.*, 5:61–67.
73. Rucker, R. R., Yasutake, W. T., and Wolf, H. (1961): Trout hepatoma—A preliminary report. *Prog. Fish-Cult.*, 23:3–7.
74. Salhab, A. S., and Edwards, G. S. (1977): Comparative *in vitro* metabolism of aflatoxicol by liver preparations from animals and humans. *Cancer Res.*, 37:1,016–1,021.
75. Sato, S., Matsushima, T., Tanaka, N., Sugimura, T., and Takashima, F. (1973): Hepatic tumors in the guppy (*Lebistes reticulatus*) induced by aflatoxin B$_1$, dimethylnitrosamine, and 2-acetylaminofluorene. *J. Natl. Cancer Inst.*, 50:765–778.
76. Scarpelli, D. G. (1967): Ultrastructural and biochemical observations in trout hepatoma. In: *Trout Hepatoma Research Conference Papers*, edited by J. E. Halver and I. A. Mitchell, Res. Rept. 70:60–71. Bureau of Sport Fisheries and Wildlife, Washington, D.C.
77. Scarpelli, D. G. (1974): Mitogenic activity of sterculic acid, a cyclopropenoid fatty acid. *Science*, 185:958–960.
78. Scarpelli, D. G. (1975): Preliminary observations on the mitogenic effect of cyclopropenoid fatty acids on rat pancreas. *Cancer Res.*, 35:2,278–2,283.
79. Scarpelli, D. G. (1976): Drug metabolism and aflatoxin-induced hepatoma in rainbow trout (*Salmo gairdneri*). *Prog. Exp. Tumor Res.*, 20:339–350.
80. Scarpelli, D. G., Lee, D. J., Sinnhuber, R. O., and Chiga, M. (1974): Cytoplasmic alterations of hepatocytes in rainbow trout (*Salmo gairdneri*) induced by cyclopropenoid fatty acids. *Cancer Res.*, 34:2,984–2,990.

81. Schoenhard, G. L., Lee, D. J., Howell, S. E., Pawlowski, N. E., Libbey, L. M., and Sinnhuber, R. O. (1976): Aflatoxin B₁ metabolism to aflatoxicol and derivatives lethal to *Bacillus subtilis* GSY 1057 by rainbow trout (*Salmo gairdneri*) liver. *Cancer Res.*, 36:2,040–2,045.
82. Schoenhard, G. L., Hendricks, J. D., Nixon, J. E., Lee, D. J., Wales, J. H., Sinnhuber, R. O. and Pawlowski, N. E. Aflatoxicol-induced hepatocellular carcinoma in rainbow trout (*Salmo gairdneri*) and the synergistic effects of cyclopropenoid fatty acids. *Cancer Res.*, 41:1,011–1,014.
83. Schoental, R. (1970): Hepatotoxic activity of retrorsine, senkirkine, and hydroxysenkirkine in newborn rats, and the role of epoxides in carcinogenesis in pyrrolizidine alkaloids and aflatoxins. *Nature*, 227:401–402.
84. Sinnhuber, R. O., Hendricks, J. D., Putnam, G. B., Wales, J. H., Pawlowski, N. E., Nixon, J. E., and Lee, D. J. (1976): Sterculic acid, a naturally occurring cyclopropene fatty acid, a liver carcinogen to rainbow trout (*Salmo gairdneri*). *Fed. Proc.*, 35:505.
85. Sinnhuber, R. O., Hendricks, J. D., Wales, J. H., and Putnam, G. B. (1977): Neoplasms in rainbow trout, a sensitive animal model for environmental carcinogenesis. *Ann. N.Y. Acad. Sci.*, 298:389–408.
86. Sinnhuber, R. O., Lee, D. J., Wales, J. H., and Ayres, J. L. (1968): Dietary factors and hepatoma in rainbow trout (*Salmo gairdneri*). II. Cocarcinogenesis by cyclopropenoid fatty acids and the effect of gossypol and altered lipids on aflatoxin-induced liver cancer. *J. Natl. Cancer Inst.*, 41:1,293–1,301.
87. Sinnhuber, R. O., Lee, D. J., Wales, J. H., Landers, M. K., and Keyl, A. C. (1974): Hepatic carcinogenesis of aflatoxin M₁ in rainbow trout (*Salmo gairdneri*) and its enhancement by cyclopropene fatty acids. *J. Natl. Cancer Inst.*, 53:1,285–1,288.
88. Sinnhuber, R. O., and Wales, J. H. (1978): The effects of mycotoxins in aquatic animals. In: *Mycotoxic Fungi, Mycotoxins, Mycotoxicoses: An Encyclopedia Handbook*, edited by T. D. Wyllie and L. G. Morehouse, pp. 489–509. Marcel Dekker Inc., New York.
89. Sinnhuber, R. O., Wales, J. H., Ayres, J. L., Engebrecht, R A., and Amend, D. L. (1968): Dietary factors and hepatoma in rainbow trout (*Salmo gairdneri*). I. Aflatoxins in vegetable protein feedstuffs. *J. Natl. Cancer Inst.*, 41:711–718.
90. Sinnhuber, R. O., Wales, J. H., Hendricks, J. D., Putnam, G. B., Nixon, J. E., and Pawlowski, N. E. (1977): Trout bioassay of mycotoxins. In: *Mycotoxins in Human and Animal Health*, edited by J. V. Rodricks, C. W. Hesseltine, and M. A. Mehlman, pp. 731–744. Pathotox Publishers, Inc., Park Forest South, Illinois.
91. Sinnhuber, R. O., Wales, J. H., and Lee, D. J. (1966): Cyclopropenoids, cocarcinogens for aflatoxin-induced hepatoma in trout. *Fed. Proc.*, 25:555.
92. Squire, R. A., and Levitt, M. H. (1975): Report of a workshop on classification of specific hepatocellular lesions in rats. *Cancer Res.*, 35:3,214–3,223.

93. Stanton, M. F. (1965): Diethylnitrosamine-induced hepatic degeneration and neoplasia in the aquarium fish *Brachydanio rerio*. *J. Natl. Cancer Inst.*, 34:117–130.

94. Stewart, H. L., Williams, G., Keysser, C. H., Lombard, L. S., and Montali, R. J. (1980): Histologic typing of liver tumors of the rat. *J. Natl. Cancer Inst.*, 64:179–206.

95. Stoloff, L., Verrett, J. M., Dantzman, J. and Reynaldo, E. F. (1972): Toxicological study of aflatoxin P$_1$ using the fertile chicken egg. *Toxicol. Appl. Pharmacol.*, 23:528–531.

96. Stott, W. T., and Sinnhuber, R. O. (1978): Trout hepatic enzyme activation of aflatoxin B$_1$ in a mutagen assay system and the inhibitory effect of PCBs. *Bull. Environ. Contam. Toxicol.*, 19:35–41.

97. Stott, W. T., and Sinnhuber, R. O. (1978): Dietary protein levels and aflatoxin B$_1$ metabolism in rainbow trout (*Salmo gairdneri*). *J. Environ. Pathol. Toxicol.* 2:379–388.

98. Stott, W. T., and Sinnhuber, R. O. (1979): Dietary casein levels and aflatoxin B$_1$ metabolism in rainbow trout (*Salmo gairdneri*). In: *Pesticide and Xenobiotic Metabolism in Aquatic Organisms*, edited by M. A. Q. Khan, J. J. Lech, and J. J. Menn, ACS Symposium Series, No. 99, pp. 389–400. American Chemical Society, Miami.

99. Struthers, B. J., Wales, J. H., Lee, D. J., and Sinnhuber, R. O. (1975): Liver composition and histology of rainbow trout fed cyclopropenoid fatty acids. *Exp. Molec. Pathol.*, 23:164–170.

100. Sugimura, T., Fugimura, S., and Baba, T. (1970): Tumor production in the glandular stomach and alimentary tract of the rat by N-methyl-N′-nitro-N-nitrosoguanidine. *Cancer Res.*, 30:455–465.

101. Swenson, D. H., Lin, J. F., Miller, E. C., and Miller, J. A. (1977): Aflatoxin B$_1$-2,3-oxide as a probable intermediate in the covalent binding of aflatoxins B$_1$ and B$_2$ to rat liver DNA and ribosomal RNA *in vivo*. *Cancer Res.*, 37:172–181.

102. Swenson, D. H., Miller, E. C., and Miller, J. A. (1974): Aflatoxin B$_1$-2,3-oxide: Evidence for its formation in rat liver *in vivo* and by human liver microsomes *in vitro*. *Biochem. Biophys. Res. Commun.*, 60:1,036–1,043.

103. Swenson, D. H., Miller, J. A., and Miller, E. C. (1973): 2,3-dihydro-2,3-dihydroxy-aflatoxin B$_1$: An acid hydrolysis product of an RNA-aflatoxin B$_1$ adduct formed by hamster and rat liver microsomes *in vitro*. *Biochem. Biophys. Res. Commun.*, 53:1,260–1,267.

104. Swenson, D. H., Miller, J. A., and Miller, E. C. (1975): The reactivity and carcinogenicity of aflatoxin B$_1$-2,3-dichloride, a model for the putative 2,3-oxide metabolite of aflatoxin B$_1$. *Cancer Res.*, 35:3,811–3,823.

105. Takashima, F. (1976): Hepatoma and cutaneous fibrosarcoma in hatchery-reared trout and salmon related to gonadal maturation. *Prog. Exp. Tumor Res.*, 20:351–366.

106. Terao, K. (1978): Mesotheliomas induced by sterigmatocystin in wistar rats. *Gann*, 69:237–247.

107. Terracini, B., Magee, P. N., and Barnes, J. M. (1967): Hepatic pathology in rats on low dietary levels of dimethylnitrosamine. *Br. J. Cancer*, 21:559–565.

108. Voss, S. D., Shelton, D. W., and Hendricks, J. D. (1972): Induction of hepatic microsomal enzymes in rainbow trout by dietary Aroclor 1254 and the effect of cyclopropenoid fatty acids. *Arch. Environ. Contam. Toxicol. (in press)*.

109. Wales, J. H. (1970): Hepatoma in rainbow trout. In: *A Symposium on Diseases of Fishes and Shellfishes*, edited by S. F. Snieszko, 5:351–365. American Fisheries Society, Washington, D. C.

110. Wales, J. H. (1979): Induction of hepatoma in rainbow trout *Salmo gairdneri* Richardson by the egg bath technique. *J. Fish Dis.*, 2:563–566.

111. Wales, J. H., and Sinnhuber, R. O. (1972): Brief communication: Hepatomas induced by aflatoxin in the sockeye salmon (*Oncorhynchus nerka*). *J. Natl. Cancer Inst.*, 48:1,529–1,530.

112. Wales, J. H., and Sinnhuber, R. O. (1973): Trout hepatoma: Fibrosis and lymphocytosis as suppressive mechanisms in the rainbow trout (*Salmo gairdneri*). *Anat. Rec.*, 175:97–106.

113. Wales, J. H., Sinnhuber, R. O., Hendricks, J. D., Nixon, J. E., and Eisele, T. A. (1978): Aflatoxin B₁ induction of hepatocellular carcinoma in the embryos of rainbow trout (*Salmo gairdneri*). *J. Natl. Cancer Inst.*, 60:1,133–1,139.

114. Wellings, S. R. (1969): Neoplasia and primitive vertebrate phylogeny: Echinoderms, prevertebrates, and fishes—A review. *Natl. Cancer Inst. Monogr.*, 31:59–128.

115. Wogan, G. N., Edwards, G. E., and Newberne, P. M. (1971): Structure-activity relationship in toxicity and carcinogenicity of aflatoxins and analogs. *Cancer Res.*, 31:1,936–1,942.

116. Wogan, G. N., and Paglialunga, S. (1974): Carcinogenicity of synthetic aflatoxin M₁ in rats. *Food Cosmet. Toxicol.*, 12:381–384.

117. Wogan, G. N., Paglialunga, S., and Newberne, P. M. (1974): Carcinogenic effects of low dietary levels of aflatoxin B₁ in rats. *Food Cosmet. Toxicol.*, 12:681–685.

118. Wolf, H., and Jackson, E. W. (1967): Hepatoma in salmonids: The role of cottonseed products and species differences. In: *Trout Hepatoma Research Conference Papers*, edited by J. E. Halver and I. A. Mitchell, Res. Rept., 70:29–33. Bureau of Sport Fisheries and Wildlife, Washington, D. C.

119. Wong, J. J., and Hsieh, D. P. H. (1976): Mutagenicity of aflatoxins related to their metabolism and carcinogenic potential. *Proc. Natl. Acad. Sci.*, 73:2,241–2,244.

120. Wong, J. J., Singh, R., and Hsieh, D. P. H. (1977): Mutagenicity of fungal metabolites related to aflatoxin synthesis. *Mutat. Res.*, 44:447–450.

# Subject Index

*213*